NUTRITION

**Recent Titles in
Health and Medical Issues Today**

Obesity
Evelyn B. Kelly

Stem Cells
Evelyn B. Kelly

Organ Transplantation
David Petechuk

Alternative Medicine
Christine A. Larson

Gene Therapy
Evelyn B. Kelly

Sports Medicine
Jennifer L. Minigh

NUTRITION

Sharon Zoumbaris

Health and Medical Issues Today

GREENWOOD PRESS
An Imprint of ABC-CLIO, LLC

A B C ☰ C L I O

Santa Barbara, California • Denver, Colorado • Oxford, England

SKOKIE PUBLIC LIBRARY

Copyright 2009 by Sharon Zoumbaris

All rights reserved. No part of this publication may be reproduced, stored in a retrieval system, or transmitted, in any form or by any means, electronic, mechanical, photocopying, recording, or otherwise, except for the inclusion of brief quotations in a review, without prior permission in writing from the publisher.

Library of Congress Cataloging-in-Publication Data

Zoumbaris, Sharon K., 1955–
  Nutrition / Sharon Zoumbaris.
      p. cm. — (Health and medical issues today)
  Includes bibliographical references and index.
  ISBN 978-0-313-34985-0 (pbk : alk. paper) — 978-0-313-34986-7 (ebook)
 1. Nutrition. 2. Nutrition—Requirements. 3. Nutrition—Genetic aspects. 4. Nutrition policy. I. Title. II. Series: Health and medical issues today.
  [DNLM: 1. Nutritional Requirements. 2. Diet. 3. Food. 4. Nurtrigenomics.
5. Nutrition Policy. QU 145 Z91n 2009]
  RA784.Z68 2009
  613.2—dc22   2009022921

13 12 11 10 9   1 2 3 4 5

This book is also available on the World Wide Web as an eBook.
Visit www.abc-clio.com for details.

ABC-CLIO, LLC
130 Cremona Drive, P.O. Box 1911
Santa Barbara, California 93116-1911

This book is printed on acid-free paper ∞

Manufactured in the United States of America

Contents

Series Foreword vii
Preface ix
Introduction xiii

Section One: Overview

1 A Brief History of Nutrition and the Future of Nutrigenomics 3
2 Basics and Principles of Nutrition and Its Practitioners 11
3 Nutrition Guidelines and the Government's Role 17

Section Two: Controversies and Issues Relating to Nutrition

4 Food Irradiation: Past Its Shelf Life? 29
5 Genetically Modified Food: Are We Playing God? 45
6 Vitamins and Supplements: A Love-Hate Relationship 65
7 Vegetarians: You Are What You Eat 77
8 Organic Food: Better or Just More Expensive? 99
9 From the Field to the Table: How Safe Is Our Food? 119
10 Bans on Fast Food and Junk Food: Who Wins, Who Loses? 143

Section Three: References and Resources

A	Annotated Primary Source Documents	159
B	Nutrition Timeline	191
C	Directory of Organizations	195

Notes	199
Glossary	207
Bibliography	213
Index	227

SERIES FOREWORD

Every day, the public is bombarded with information on developments in medicine and health care. Whether they involve the latest techniques in treatments or research, or concerns over public health threats, these developments directly impact the lives of people more than almost any other issue. Although there are many sources for understanding these topics—from Web sites and blogs to newspapers and magazines—students and ordinary citizens often need a single resource that makes sense of the complex health and medical issues affecting their daily lives.

The *Health and Medical Issues Today* series provides just such a one-stop resource for obtaining a solid overview of the most controversial areas of contemporary health care. Each volume addresses one topic and provides a balanced summary of what is known. These volumes offer an excellent first step for students and laypeople interested in understanding how health care works in our society today.

Each volume is broken into several sections to provide readers and researchers with easy access to the information they need:

- Section I provides overview chapters on background information that a citizen needs to intelligently understand the topic—including chapters on such areas as the historical, scientific, medical, social, and legal issues involved.
- Section II provides capsule examinations of the most heated contemporary issues and debates, and analyzes in a balanced manner the viewpoints held by various advocates in the debates.

- Section III provides a selection of reference material, such as annotated primary source documents, a timeline of important events, and a directory of organizations that serve as the best next step in learning about the topic at hand.

The *Health and Medical Issues Today* series strives to provide readers with all the information needed to begin making sense of some of the most important contemporary debates. The series includes volumes on such topics as stem-cell research, obesity, gene therapy, alternative medicine, organ transplantation, mental health, and more.

PREFACE

Proper nutrition is an elusive goal for many Americans. Thanks to the mass appeal of fast food, the hectic lifestyle of many families, and the overwhelming amount of conflicting information streamed to consumers daily, too few people eat a healthy diet. The intent of this book is to offer a roadmap through the confusing and controversial aspects of nutrition. Although the subjects—from food irradiation to a government ban on fast food and junk food—are not new to consumers, it is important to fully understand the latest research, statistics, and developments in each. This information is of great importance to every American, because food is a basic necessity for every living creature. This book is intended to provide key knowledge to assist readers as they work to understand the realities of the food they eat: how it is grown, processed, and treated, and what that means for healthy nutrition.

Chapter 1, "A Brief History of Nutrition and the Future of Nutrigenomics," describes the early science of nutrition. This section introduces problems Americans face such as a growing obesity rate and unhealthy food choices, and examines how national eating habits have been influenced over time. The chapter begins with a look at how pioneering individuals unraveled the mystery of nutrition, and ends with a look at the future of research in nutrigenomics—the study of how food affects our genes and how unique genetic differences change the way an individual assimilates nutrients.

Chapter 2, "Basics and Principles of Nutrition and Its Practitioners," provides a clear understanding of human nutrition. This chapter offers readers a simple breakdown of the six essential nutrient categories needed for healthy nutrition, as well as other key ingredients for physical health.

There is also a discussion of careers in the field of human nutrition, from registered dietitians to food scientists.

Chapter 3, "Nutrition Guidelines and the Government's Role," describes the alphabet soup of federal agencies now measuring and regulating our food from the field to the table. Government agencies were set up initially to promote the business of American agriculture, and later to determine the nutritional value of foods and to monitor food safety. The chapter also illustrates how the U.S. government offers nutrition education to the American public through dietary guidelines and other publications and programs.

Chapter 4, "Food Irradiation: Past Its Shelf Life?" examines the process as well as the pros and cons of treating food using radiation to prevent illness, eliminate insects, and increase the shelf life of fresh and processed foods. Manufacturers have been treating U.S. food with ionizing radiation for decades, but questions still remain about long-term safety, nutrient losses, and possible chemical changes in irradiated food. The chapter looks at consumer reactions to irradiated food, the history of the U.S. government's role in the industry, and the debate over current regulations and required labels.

Chapter 5, "Genetically Modified Food: Are We Playing God?" takes a close look at the history of genetically modified (GM) organisms, the questions associated with their use, and the pros and cons of GM crops. It details the early days of GM technology, and how critics and supporters view the future. The chapter also presents both sides of the debate over perceived environmental hazards, human health risks, and long-term economic effects.

Chapter 6, "Vitamins and Supplements: A Love-Hate Relationship," compares the hype about vitamins and supplements to the facts. The chapter looks at new research, and presents opposing points of view concerning the overall effects of vitamins and supplements on health. Details of government warnings are also included.

Chapter 7, "Vegetarians: You Are What You Eat," looks at the American love affair with meat, as well as new statistics on why some Americans are turning to meatless eating. The health benefits of a vegetarian diet, and the environmental effects of livestock production, offer readers food for thought.

Chapter 8, "Organic Food: Better or Just More Expensive?" details the benefits and costs of buying and eating organic food. The chapter describes the history of the organic movement and the issues and controversies dividing the industry, from food safety to global warming. For consumers not familiar with various labels—everything from "USDA

PREFACE

organic" to "free-range" and "cage-free"—this chapter explains the differences along with pertinent government regulations.

Chapter 9, "From the Field to the Table: How Safe Is Our Food?" offers a view of U.S. food safety, including the impact of foodborne illness as well as risks from irradiation, genetically modified foods, additives such as growth hormones, and problems with imported foods. This chapter explains how key outbreaks of food poisoning in the United States shaped government food safety regulations, and how complicated checks and balances shared by several federal agencies continue to influence the food industry, the government, and consumer groups. Important rules for providing food safety at home are included, along with a look at the organizations working to keep food industry lobbyists in check.

Chapter 10, "Bans on Fast Food and Junk Food: Who Wins, Who Loses?" examines the government's role in restricting access to fast food and junk food. This newest weapon in an arsenal of methods to improve national nutrition and to educate Americans about healthy eating is considered heavy-handed by opponents, and a welcome tool by supporters.

Appendix A consists of annotated primary source documents that contain fundamental nutrition information. They comprise the 1906 Pure Food and Drug Act; an example of the DASH (Dietary Approaches to Stop Hypertension) Eating Plan; a guide to the updated Nutrition Facts Label; a look at FDA irradiation regulations on shell eggs; basic labeling information for the National Organic Program; an FDA list of questions and answers on foodborne illness; an FDA background document on the food safety system known as Hazard Analysis and Critical Control Point, or HACCP; an outline of the National School Lunch Program; and sample menus for a 2000-calorie food plan.

Appendix B is a timeline of important moments in the history of nutrition, ranging from the discovery of cures for diseases such as scurvy to the 2008 fast-food moratorium passed by the Los Angeles City Council. Appendix C is a directory of organizations useful for further research. A comprehensive glossary and bibliography conclude the volume.

The author and publisher of this volume do not endorse, recommend, or make representations with respect to the research, services, medication, treatments, or products mentioned herein. Nothing in the book is intended as a substitute for medical advice. For information about personal circumstances, consult a physician or other health care professional.

INTRODUCTION

There is no miracle cure for what ails Americans nutritionally. The answer is surprisingly simple and includes these suggestions: eat a variety of fresh, healthy foods that include healthy fats, complex carbohydrates, protein, vegetables, and fruits; avoid a diet heavy in processed foods that contain high levels of sodium, saturated fats, trans fats, sugar, or other sweeteners or additives; sit down for meals rather than eating in the car or on the run; drink plenty of water; and exercise.

This information has always been available to Americans, but over the decades the message has been masked by the siren song of convenient, cheap, quick food options. Unfortunately, as consumers moved away from preparing their own meals, they also moved away from knowledge of basic nutrition. Now, confronted with soaring food prices, global grain shortages, and new, antibiotic-resistant bacteria, consumers face difficult and sometimes dangerous food choices. Practices Americans previously avoided, such as irradiating meat to kill bacteria, are getting a fresh look. In Europe, concerns about price and supply have even overruled opposition to genetically modified foods, which Europeans originally labeled Frankenfoods.

In these changing times, it is more important than ever to be educated about food, how it was prepared, and where it originated. Those old enough to remember the 1970s will find the world's current food issues reminiscent of that time, when supplies dropped as high energy costs pushed up food prices and droughts and other major weather events destroyed crops. Climate change plays a role in present concerns about international food supply, but another major factor is an expanding middle class in countries such as China and India. In these countries, hundreds of millions of people, now earning larger incomes, have created unprecedented demand for expensive meats and other costly imports. This demand makes growing for the wealthy a better business choice than growing for the masses.

For decades, Americans have moved away from manual labor and farming, leaving it to fewer and fewer people to cultivate our nation's food supply. Small farmers have trouble competing with large agribusiness operations and have seen their profits shrink. In fact, a large percentage of every U.S. food dollar goes not to the farmers but to the food processors, marketers, and transporters who handle the food after it leaves the farm. The resurgence in organic farming, on the other hand, now focuses on the interdependence of humans and nature, and is seen by supporters as a way to sustain the people who grow our nation's food. As government applies new laws to help consumers make good food decisions, Americans are struggling with the difficult choices they face.

This book is a guide to help readers understand food and healthy nutrition. It will provide answers to the question, "What should we eat?" Our national ignorance of nutrition and our demand for heavily processed food have been linked to skyrocketing obesity rates, diet-related diseases, and a food production system heavily dependent on shrinking supplies of petroleum. Americans live in the land of freedom and can choose whatever they want—from organic food, vegetarian meals, meat treated with irradiation, genetically modified foods, or fast food to vitamins and supplements. At the very least, the choice should be an informed one.

Section One

Overview

CHAPTER 1

A Brief History of Nutrition and the Future of Nutrigenomics

Nutrition is the science of how the human body uses food. But nutrition today is more than science—it is also politics. The food industry generates more than one trillion dollars in annual sales. This means that what we eat is influenced by big business, government policy, and profits, as well as by geography, climate, economics, and culture. Nowhere is this more evident than in America, where we have changed from a nation with an honest appetite to an obedient market for cheap, fast food.

Eating is one of life's necessities. In many cultures, it is also one of life's pleasures. Unfortunately, in today's America hardly anyone seems concerned with the flavor or authenticity of our food; it is the speed and packaging that get all the attention. As Americans settle for convenience over nutrition, more than ever food is filled with antibiotics, laden with fats, saturated with high-fructose corn syrup, and loaded with salt. Even fruits and vegetables are a far cry from fresh. They are grown, packaged, and shipped from all corners of the globe, bringing with them a huge energy and transportation price tag. On average, each food item in a typical U.S. meal has traveled 1,500 miles.[1] Overall, the energy calories consumed by producing, packaging, and shipping the food far outweigh the energy calories consumed by simply eating it.

Our national obesity rate is linked to increasing rates of hypertension, heart disease, and diabetes. Tragically, children of the present generation face a shorter life expectancy than their parents. If it is clear that what we eat affects our health, why do Americans make such poor food choices? Why don't we separate what's good from what's bad? Perhaps it is because advertisers bombard us with commercials filled with hungry people devouring hamburgers, guzzling soft drinks, and inhaling huge amounts of cheap, processed food. Or maybe it is due to the newspapers, television programs, and magazines that routinely serve up contradictory nutritional studies, fueling controversies and raising questions.

The answer to our nutritional dilemma may come from new discoveries using nutritional genomics, or "nutrigenomics"—the study of how different foods affect genes and how genetic differences may change the way nutrients are processed. Or it may be found in simple, commonsense tips: take smaller bites or portions; don't snack between meals; eat a variety of fresh and healthy fruits, vegetables, protein, fats, and complex carbohydrates; eat sitting down to a meal rather than in the car or on the run; savor a meal slowly rather than eating in front of the television. Whatever the solutions may be, it's important to first understand how the science of nutrition evolved.

EARLY HISTORY

Humankind has struggled with food since Adam and Eve took a bite of the apple. History includes various nutritional theories dating back to the ancient Greeks. Around 500 B.C., the philosopher Anaxagoras suggested that nutrition was based on the fact that everything contained small amounts of everything else. He believed that in order for food to turn into bone, hair, or flesh, it must already contain all of those properties within it. Hippocrates, in the fourth century B.C., had different ideas about nutrition. He suggested that food was the body's best medicine. Although his gentle approach to health and diet was the genesis of today's Hippocratic Oath, his suggested link between diet and disease was not widely embraced. Instead, the ancient Greeks favored the theory that matter was composed of four elements—earth, air, fire, and water—and the body needed to be balanced in all four to remain healthy.

It wasn't until the late 1500s that Belgian physician Johannes Baptista van Helmont sought to discredit the ancient Greek theory that all matter is composed of the four elements. To prove his point, he launched an experiment to see whether plants absorbed soil as they grew, and found that there was no change in the amount of soil. This experiment was a breakthrough in methodology. It represented the first application of quantitative methods to a biological question, and earned van Helmont the label "Father of Biochemistry."[2] Van Helmont opened the door to scientific analysis. Other scientists followed, although breakthroughs at first were few and far between.

An exciting link in the connection between diet and health was discovered in 1747 by James Lind, a British naval surgeon. Lind conducted shipboard experiments to unravel the mystery of scurvy, a serious nutritional disorder now known to be caused by a lack of vitamin C. Symptoms include extreme fatigue, nausea, muscle and joint pain, and internal bleeding. As a scientist in the age of exploration, Lind knew only too well the devastating effects of scurvy on sailors. As he treated sick sailors, he kept all factors the same except one: he gave each man a daily dose of a different remedy. His choices for treatment were cider, vinegar, sea water, oranges, or lemons. Those men given the oranges and lemons quickly improved. The men given hard cider, which contains some vitamin C, also showed improvement. Thanks to treatment with vitamin C based on Lind's early research, scurvy is no longer a health threat. Lind is credited with establishing the first clinical trial. He published his results in a book titled *A Treatise of the Scurvy* (1753). Lind's work clearly showed other scientists the importance of diet in treating and preventing disease.

In 1897, a Dutch physician named Christian Eijkman attempted to unravel the causes of beriberi, a nutritional disease that affects the nerves, digestive system, and heart. Working with rice, he discovered that something important was lost when the hulls where removed and the rice was polished. The missing nutrient, thiamine—a B vitamin—was not present in the polished grains. Soon afterward, Frederick Gowland Hopkins, a British biochemist interested in the puzzle of nutritional-deficiency diseases, shared the 1929 Nobel Prize in physiology and medicine with Eijkman for their research on vitamins. Hopkins's early investigations, published in 1906, were based on diets he created for experimental animals. He concluded that even when diets appeared adequate, there were "accessory food factors" that were essential for growth and good health. His two papers on the subject, published in 1906 and 1912, are considered the first explanations of the concept of vitamins.[3] His experiments are considered classics in the history of nutrition. His work led other researchers to identify the fat-soluble and water-soluble vitamins.

At the same time, a Polish American biochemist named Casimir Funk published a paper in 1912 on diseases caused by vitamin deficiencies. He developed the term "vitamine," from which "vitamin" is derived. The word *vita* is Latin for life, and "amine" was added because Funk believed the substances were part of a special group of chemicals known as amines. In his paper, Funk named four vitamins—B1 or thiamine, B2, C, and D—as factors necessary to prevent disease and maintain good health. The "e" on the end of "vitamine" was dropped when scientists discovered that not all vitamins contain an amine group.

NINETEENTH-CENTURY ADVANCES

In the nineteenth century, scientists interested in human nutrition broadened their focus from vitamins to the study of how the body processes and synthesizes food. In 1842, a German physician, Julius Robert von Mayer, calculated the amount of heat produced by compressing gases. His principle was then applied to the heat or energy given off when food was eaten. This led to the practice of measuring "food energy" in calories. Calories are used by the body during metabolism, the process by which food is broken down and transformed into nutrients or other simple elements used by the body. A calorie is the amount of heat necessary to raise the temperature of a kilogram of water 1°C at normal atmospheric pressure.

Von Mayer worked closely with Baron Justus von Liebig, an early leader in biochemistry who studied the link between chemical science and food, nutrition, and agriculture. Von Liebig was born in Germany in 1803 and died in 1873. His work focused on the theory that body heat and the ability of muscles to do work came from the energy derived from fats and carbohydrates. These nutrition pioneers learned that food was the key to providing the human body with energy. At the same time, research continued on the properties of food itself. American chemist Lafayette Benedict Mendel partnered with Thomas B. Osborne to break new ground in the understanding of nutrients. The two devised experiments in which they fed rats a controlled diet and measured the food intake and the changes in each animal's weight. The men were following the lead of another biochemist, Elmer McCollum, known for using rats for experiments and testing. They also discovered a variety of substances necessary for a healthy diet.

McCollum was the first scientist to use rat colonies to examine nutritional diseases. In 1912, he realized that rats fed a diet deficient in certain fats quickly improved and resumed normal growth once the fats were reintroduced. This led to the first discovery of a fat-soluble nutrient, which McCollum named vitamin A. Mendel and Osborne discovered vitamin A just a few weeks later. McCollum went on to prove that a different water-soluble substance, which he named vitamin B, was also necessary for good health. At the same time, Mendel and Osborne were doing their own experiments with vitamin B and other key nutrients. They also established that the human body cannot produce all the nutrients it needs on its own and must get those elements through food.

McCollum is best known for his research producing rickets in lab rats. Rickets is a disease of poor nutrition. Symptoms include bending, fractures, and swelling in the ends of the long bones in the leg. McCollum was able to isolate the missing nutrient in the rats' diets, which he named vitamin D. Vitamin D aids in the absorption of calcium, which is needed for the formation of bones and teeth. Vitamin D is also formed in the body when a person is exposed to sunlight. McCollum's book *The Newer Knowledge of Nutrition* (1918) influenced a new era in nutrition. Study and research began to focus on identification and isolation of vitamins and essential nutrients.

Vitamin deficiencies were such a major cause of poor health in the late 1800s that the U.S. government, led by W. O. Atwater, sought ways to improve nutrition. Atwater worked with the Connecticut legislature to establish the first state agricultural station in the United States. He was first introduced to early European agricultural experiment stations while studying in Germany. The U.S. government's interest in nutrition and disease prevention was due in part to the massive deaths of soldiers during the Civil War. Medical records from the war showed that for every soldier killed in battle or dead of wounds, two died of disease brought on by poor sanitation, inadequate diet and nutrition, and overall poor health.[4] The government's efforts, driven by those 380,000 unnecessary deaths, focused on improving the nutrition of all Americans.

In 1888, Atwater was named the first director of the Office of Experiment Stations of the U.S. Department of Agriculture (USDA). Under his guidance, the earliest in a long history of dietary guidelines for Americans was published. Then, in May of 1894, Congress approved an agricultural appropriations bill of $10,000 for food investigations. This was the first federal funding of human nutrition research in the United States. It was a welcome victory for Atwater, the son of a Methodist minister whose doctoral thesis at Yale was an analysis of feed corn.

Atwater's research continued throughout his life, and focused on issues such as the effects of cooking and food processing on the nutritional quality of food, and the amounts and types of nutrients people need to function at their best. In 1892, Atwater partnered with E. B. Rosa, professor of physics at Wesleyan University, to build the Atwater-Rosa calorimeter. It took five years to complete, and provided new and better information about calories and nutrients. Atwater went on to prepare elaborate tables giving the caloric value of many foods. Atwater's tables were published in 1896, and much of his data is still in use today.

DIETITIANS

In 1896, Atwater and A. P. Bryant published *The Chemical Composition of American Food Materials*, known simply as *Bulletin No. 28*. This document, considered the dietitian's bible, listed the minimum, maximum, and average values of the known nutrients in all American foods that had been analyzed by July 1895. A 1906 reprinting of the bulletin stood virtually unchanged until 1940, when an updated version was published.

In fact, Atwater was not the only scientist bringing a new urgency to the field of nutrition. Several notable American women emerged in the 1930s and made major contributions. Adelle Davis and Flemmie Pansy Kittrell were both born in 1904—Davis in Indiana and Kittrell in North Carolina—and each woman gained international recognition for her strong views on the link between nutrition and health. Kittrell was the first African American woman to earn a PhD in nutrition. She graduated from Hampton Institute in Virginia with an undergraduate degree in science in 1928. With the encouragement of her professors, she enrolled at Cornell University.

There were few blacks in higher education during that time, but Kittrell was not intimidated, and in 1938 she was awarded her PhD in nutrition with honors. Kittrell was deeply affected by a nutritional survey she completed in the West African nation of Liberia. In 1947, she began a lifelong program of international activism. Kittrell worked tirelessly to draw needed attention to the nutrition of African children.

Davis began her nutrition training at Purdue University in Lafayette in 1923, but after two years transferred to the University of California at Berkeley, where she received a BA degree in dietetics in 1927 and earned the nickname "Vitamin Davis" from her fellow students.[5] At that time, UC Berkeley was thought to be the top research institution in the United States in the study of vitamins. Davis was constantly talking about her beliefs that vitamins, taken in sufficient quantities, could improve mood, increase energy, extend life, and ensure perfect health. Unfortunately, due to the Great Depression, many ordinary people were lucky to get enough food to eat, and there was little interest in vitamins.

In 1939, Davis received a master's degree in biochemistry from the University of Southern California School of Medicine. That year, she published a booklet and began a practice as a consulting nutritionist. Before long, Davis was quoted in the media, and she eventually succeeded in publishing several nutrition books.

In her first major publication, *Let's Cook It Right* (1947), Davis sought to educate readers. She preached the gospel of whole grains and breads, fresh vegetables, vitamins, and limits on sugar, and warned against packaged, processed foods. The 1960s and 1970s saw her fame grow as she worked tirelessly to make people aware of her version of the science of nutrition. In her book *Let's Get Well* (1965), Davis blasted advertising's role in what she called the country's nutritional decline. She continued to suggest that vitamins could determine whether a person was grouchy or cheerful, homely or beautiful. She recommended extra niacin to reduce grumpiness, and even suggested that vitamin B3 would cure schizophrenia.[6]

Many in the medical community considered Davis's ideas dangerous, and worried that people would ignore symptoms of serious disease or treat their health problems with vitamins and wheat germ. These fears were never realized, but American consumers were influenced by Davis's views. At the time of her death from cancer in 1974, *The Washington Post* reported that her four books on nutrition had sold more than 10 million copies. Nutrition advocates such as Davis were determined to educate average consumers. Unfortunately, because the science did not support her strong views, Davis ended up adding to the confusion about good nutrition.

NUTRIGENOMICS AND THE FUTURE

Today, new generations of biologists are working to define good nutrition. They have also embraced the idea of individual nutrition, giving a futuristic twist to the concept of personal nutrition. Nutrigenomics is the study of how foods affect our genes and how individual genetic differences affect the way our bodies process nutrients. Those involved with nutrigenomics believe that the information will ultimately prevent nutritional deficiencies. For example, consider the question of how many cups of coffee you should drink per day. Genetic tests can determine whether you have a specific genetic variation that makes it hard to absorb calcium in the presence of caffeine. Or consider the question, is a high-fat diet damaging to your health? Scientists now know that about 15 percent of people are born with a form of liver enzyme that causes their good cholesterol to go down in response to dietary fat. This is opposite of what should happen when dietary fat is eaten: in most people the HDL or good cholesterol level goes up.

This area of research is new, but the field is growing rapidly. There are companies already offering testing for a limited number of gene–nutrient interactions. Testing kits, available in some supermarket pharmacies and online, have users swab the inside of the cheek then send the sample and a questionnaire about diet and lifestyle back to the company's laboratories. Within weeks, a computerized analysis arrives offering highlights of the genetic test results. Yet there is still work to be done to figure out how all the genetic variables in humans relate to health and disease. Add the fact that food is full of hundreds of bioactive compounds, each influenced by where plants are grown or how and where animals are raised, and it is clear that nutrigenomics is in its infancy. But the fantasy of a personalized set of dietary guidelines is tantalizing to those with a family history of chronic disease or weight management issues.

The International Food Information Council surveyed consumer attitudes in 2005, and determined that 71 percent of Americans favor the idea of using genetic information to improve their nutrition. Another 70 percent of those surveyed were interested in learning more about how genetic information can help improve their diets and overall health. That's impressive given that only 11 percent of American adults consume the USDA recommended daily portions of fruits and vegetables. Maybe Hippocrates was right when he wrote, "Leave your drugs in the chemist's pot if you can heal the patient with food."

Chapter 2

Basics and Principles of Nutrition and Its Practitioners

At its most basic level, nutrition is the process by which we take in food, food provides energy, and energy powers the body and keeps us alive. There are six groups of essential dietary elements, called nutrients, required for a body to remain healthy. These nutrients provide energy, help us grow, and allow us to repair damaged tissues. They include proteins, carbohydrates, fats, vitamins, minerals, and water.

Proteins

Proteins are made up of chemicals called amino acids. There are 22 different amino acids; the body can make 13, but the other 9 must come from the food we eat. All amino acids contain carbon, oxygen, nitrogen, and hydrogen. The main work of proteins is to grow and repair body tissue such as bones, skin, and organs. Proteins make up much of your muscles and organs, and even some hormones. Proteins also make up hemoglobin, the part of the red blood cells that carries oxygen around the body. Finally, proteins provide a small source of energy. Humans get the protein they need from animal or plant foods, including meat, chicken, fish, eggs, nuts, dairy products, and legumes.

Carbohydrates

Carbohydrates provide energy needed for the brain, central nervous system, and muscle cells. Carbohydrates are an often misunderstood nutrient, but they are the biggest source of energy for the human body. They come in two forms, simple and complex. The simple carbohydrates, including sugars such as glucose and fructose, are quickly digested and used for immediate energy. Simple carbohydrates can be found in white potatoes, white rice, and foods made with white, refined flour. Complex carbohydrates—starches and glycogen—take longer to digest, and provide a slow but steady supply of energy. Complex carbohydrates are found in whole-grain breads, cereals, and pasta, as well as grains such as bulgur and brown rice.

FATS

The various types of fats continue to confuse American consumers. Fats come in three varieties—saturated, monounsaturated, and polyunsaturated fats—and, like carbohydrates, they contain carbon, oxygen, and hydrogen. Basically, different fats get their names from their patterns of hydrogen atoms. All fatty acids, which make up fats, contain chains of carbon atoms, with hydrogen atoms attached to some or all of the carbon atoms. These fatty acids differ in the amount of hydrogen they contain.

In carbon chains in which the carbon atoms are bonded to the maximum number of hydrogen atoms—that is, "saturated" with hydrogens—the carbon atoms are linked to each other only by single bonds. Conversely, in an "unsaturated" carbon chain, with carbon atoms bonded to fewer hydrogens, some carbon atoms are linked to each other by double bonds. The more double bonds, the fewer hydrogen molecules. Fats with one double bond are called monounsaturated; those with two or more double bonds are called polyunsaturated. Both monounsaturated and polyunsaturated fats are considered good fats by nutritionists. The monounsaturated and polyunsaturated fats found in olive oil, other vegetable oils, nuts, and fish are considered part of a healthy diet. These fats provide the high-density lipoprotein (HDL) cholesterol that protects artery walls by carrying away low-density lipoprotein (LDL), or "bad," cholesterol.

Saturated fats are found in whole milk, red meats, and other animal products, as well as in palm oil and processed foods such as margarine and pastries. These fats lack double bonds between their carbon atoms, and encourage the body to make more LDL cholesterol. LDL cholesterol, considered the harmful type of cholesterol, damages artery linings and forms deposits on artery walls. Nutritional studies clearly link saturated fats and cholesterol in the diet to increased blood cholesterol levels and a greater risk of heart attack, heart disease, stroke, and other health problems. However, nutritionists caution that it is important to have some fat in a healthy diet. Healthy, unsaturated fats build cell membranes and store the fat-soluble vitamins A, D, E, and K. Most importantly, fats are the body's most concentrated sources of energy, and take longer than proteins or carbohydrates to digest.

Trans Fats

Trans fats or trans fatty acids are just about everywhere in the typical American diet. Created through a process called hydrogenation that turns liquid oils into stick margarines or shortening, they are used to increase the shelf life and stability of processed foods. Trans fats are found in many crackers, cookies, and doughnuts, to name just a few snack foods. There is a growing concern among scientists and nutritionists that, gram for gram, trans fats are more damaging than saturated fat. In other words, French fries cooked in partially hydrogenated vegetable shortening have as much artery-clogging potential as potatoes fried in lard or beef fat. In 2006, the U.S. Food and Drug Administration (FDA) added trans fat to the nutrition label requirements established by the National Labeling and Education Act (NLEA) of 1990. Now, food manufacturers must list trans fatty acids or trans fat if a food includes at least 0.5 grams of trans fat.

VITAMINS

There are 13 vitamins needed by the body for normal growth, digestion, and resistance to infection. They also assist the body in utilizing carbohydrates, fats, and proteins more efficiently. Vitamins are found naturally in many foods, and come in two forms, fat-soluble and water-soluble. The fat-soluble vitamins, A, D, E, and K, are dissolved and stored in fats, meaning that they remain in the body longer than the water-soluble vitamins. The water-soluble vitamins, C and the eight B-complex vitamins, are dissolved and stored in water. This means they pass quickly through our bodies and must be replenished on a regular basis.

Overall, our bodies need varying amounts of vitamins to prevent vitamin deficiency diseases such as scurvy and rickets. Fifty-two percent of Americans take dietary supplements and vitamins in an attempt to compensate for their poor eating habits or other perceived nutritional deficiencies, according to an October 2007 survey by the Council for Responsible Nutrition.[1] Others rely on foods that are enriched with vitamins. For example, milk and milk products are enriched with vitamin A and often with vitamin D. Vitamins are also found naturally in a variety of foods.

Vitamin A is found in fruits, and in dark green or deep yellow and orange vegetables such as carrots, pumpkins, and spinach. It is linked to improved vision and healthy skin. "Vitamin B" refers to a group of vitamins, comprising

B1, B2, B6, and B12 as well as niacin, folic acid, biotin, and pantothenic acid. The B vitamins are involved in making the red blood cells that carry oxygen throughout the body. Folic acid, one of the B vitamins, is thought to lower the risk of neural-tube birth defects such as spina bifida. In 1996, the FDA introduced a requirement that folic acid be added to white "enriched" flour to raise the average intake for consumers. A decade later, scientists are looking at the impact of high folic acid intake on cancer. Sources of vitamin B include fish, beef, pork, chicken, whole wheat grains, green leafy vegetables, enriched breads and cereals, and dried beans.

Vitamin C helps build bones and muscles and improves some infection-fighting capabilities, but large quantities can result in kidney problems. Good sources of vitamin C include citrus fruits, strawberries, melons, sweet potatoes, cabbage, tomatoes, and broccoli.

Vitamin D plays an important role in building strong healthy bones and teeth, and also assists the body in absorbing calcium. Along with its addition to foods such as milk and orange juice, vitamin D can be found in egg yolks and fish, and is also synthesized in the body after exposure to sunshine.

Vitamin E is found in vegetable oils, dark green vegetables, nuts, poultry, seafood, and wheat germ. It helps form red blood cells, muscles, and other tissues. Vitamin K is essential for effective blood clotting. It is found in dark green vegetables, whole grains, potatoes, cabbage, and cheese.

MINERALS

Minerals come from the foods we eat, both plants and plant-eating animals. Our bodies need 21 minerals; 7 of these are considered major minerals, and 14 are called trace minerals. They all contribute to a healthy body in many ways, from regulating chemical reactions, to building bones and teeth, to making hemoglobin in red blood cells. The major minerals comprise sodium, calcium, potassium, magnesium, phosphorus, chloride, and sulfur. Well-known trace minerals include iron, iodine, zinc, manganese, selenium, chromium, and fluorine.

WATER

Finally, water is the most important nutrient of all. We need over 2 quarts of water per day to function. The exact amount needed depends on many factors, including activity levels, temperature, and humidity. A person can live for several weeks without food and other nutrients, but cannot survive for more than one week without water. Even though water does not supply any energy, it does other important work. It makes up part of our blood, cools our bodies, and carries waste away as urine. We drink water, but we also get up to 20 percent of our water from the foods we eat.

CAREERS IN NUTRITION

"Registered dietitian" is the most recognized career in the nutrition field. A registered dietitian is someone who has earned a bachelor's degree in nutrition, finished a period of supervised practice, and passed a registration examination. Registered dietitians work in four basic settings, comprising clinical, community, management, and consultant dietetics. In a clinical setting, registered dietitians will consult with doctors and other health care professionals and provide services for patients in hospitals or senior care facilities. They develop nutrition programs, evaluate the results, and continually assess patients' needs.

Those who work in nutrition management often oversee large-scale food service systems in company cafeterias, prisons, health care facilities, or schools. They handle the budget and the purchase of food, and enforce sanitary and safety regulations. People with advanced degrees in nutrition and food science also conduct research projects for business, industry, health care institutions, and the government. These experts may investigate the effect of diet on health, or help develop food products.

A number of registered dietitians offer personal nutrition counseling directly to the public. For those not interested in private practice, there are growing opportunities in new areas working with supermarkets, professional sports teams, and other businesses, as well as in traditional settings in home health agencies, public health clinics, and hospitals.

The work of agricultural and food scientists also plays a key role in maintaining the nation's nutrition by ensuring both productivity and the safety of the food supply. Agricultural science is a discipline closely related to biology. Every day these scientists are discovering new food sources, and analyzing food to determine its vitamin, fat, protein, and sugar content. They look for ways to improve crop yields, to control pests, and to manipulate the genetic materials of some plants to make them more disease-resistant or productive. They also develop new methods for the processing, preservation, packaging, and storage of food according to industry and government regulations.

CHAPTER 3

Nutrition Guidelines and the Government's Role

Soaring fuel prices, global grain shortages, and massive food recalls are putting new pressures on the U.S. government and its role in the nation's food and nutrition. Throughout U.S. history, the government has regulated food in an effort to ensure its quality and safety. The bulk of federal legislation began with the 1906 Pure Food and Drug Act, and today the U.S. Food and Drug Administration regulates from one-fifth to one-quarter of U.S. gross domestic product.[1] From an economic point of view, this is a huge job for the government, and one that it has managed with varying degrees of success. Still, every American should be familiar with the Food Guide Pyramid, the Recommended Dietary Allowances (RDA), and the alphabet soup of agencies that measure and regulate food products and educate the nation about them.

HISTORY OF GOVERNMENT REGULATIONS

From their inception, government regulatory agencies were established in part to help determine the nutritional value of foods, something not always obvious to consumers. Beginning in colonial times, most food regulation in America was placed at the state and local level. But as the country grew, so did the perception that more monitoring of what was grown and sold to consumers was needed. Although nearly every agency in the federal government has something to do with food or nutrition, the two most important are the U.S. Department of Agriculture (USDA) and the Department of Health and Human Services (HHS).

President Abraham Lincoln established the Department of Agriculture in May of 1862, just a year after the start of the Civil War. However, he decided against including it in his cabinet. In 1889, President Grover Cleveland elevated the USDA to a cabinet-level department and named Norman J. Colman the new Secretary of Agriculture. Colman was born and raised on a farm in Otsego County, New York. He served with the Missouri militia during the Civil War, and was subsequently elected to the Missouri House of Representatives and then to the lieutenant governorship of Missouri. Colman then served as U.S. Commissioner of Agriculture from 1885 until 1889, when he was chosen by President Cleveland to head the USDA.

The chief responsibility of the USDA is to serve two groups: American farmers and consumers. The department assists farmers by promoting the sale and consumption of U.S. agricultural products. It serves consumers through its decisions on nutrition policy, and by safeguarding the food supply using inspections and regulatory programs.

HHS includes several smaller agencies that deal with food and nutrition, including the Food and Drug Administration (FDA), the Centers for Disease Control and Prevention (CDC), and the National Institutes of Health (NIH). The FDA regulates the safety and labeling of food products; the CDC provides research and programs to prevent diet-related diseases; and the NIH sponsors research on many other aspects of nutrition and health. Of these three small agencies, the FDA has had the biggest impact on food safety, food regulation, and overall nutrition in twentieth-century America.

THE FDA AND PUBLIC HEALTH

The FDA's mission statement, summarized by its Office of Public Affairs on its Web site, explains that the agency's primary responsibilities are to "promote and protect the public health by helping safe and effective products reach the market in a timely way, and monitoring products for continued safety after they are in use. Our work is a blending of law and science aimed at protecting consumers."[2] The FDA reviews new food products before they can be sold. It also reviews and limits the health claims that can be made on food labels. The information on current food labels is one of the most important sources of data for consumers, and is based on a long history of successful consumer legislation pushed by the FDA and consumer advocates.

First known as the Division of Chemistry, the FDA grew from comprising one chemist in 1862 to a current staff of over 9,000 employees stationed in more than 150 field offices and laboratories across the country. Today it has jurisdiction over food, human and animal drugs, medical devices, radiation-emitting products for consumers, genetically engineered food, cosmetics, and animal feed. On any given day, FDA employees evaluate applications for new human drugs, medical devices, food and color additives, infant formulas, and animal drugs. The FDA inspectors visit more than 16,000 facilities a year.

The early days in the Division of Chemistry were quiet, but with the arrival of chief chemist Harvey Washington Wiley in 1883, the agency grabbed headlines across the nation. The new chief wasted no time going after suspected food and drug frauds. Wiley, the son of an Indiana farmer, had served in the Union Army during the Civil War, had received a medical degree, and was a professor of chemistry at Purdue University. Once he became chief chemist, Wiley immediately expanded the department's research capabilities, and published *Bulletin No. 13: Foods and Food Adulterants (1887–1889)*. Wiley's actions focused media attention on dangerous products such as Banbar, a supposed cure for diabetes; Lash Lure, an eyelash dye that blinded many women; and additives such as arsenic, strychnine, and dinitrophenol—a derivative of benzene that was commonly used in the synthesis of different color dyes. In 1901, Wiley's Division of Chemistry was renamed the Bureau of Chemistry.

POISON SQUAD

Wiley made new headlines in 1902 with his "poison squad." He recruited 20 healthy young men to act as human guinea pigs by testing different food additives. When the squad's test results were released to the public in 1904, the news shocked the nation. For two years, squad members ate and drank countless questionable foods to determine whether preservatives, color additives, dyes, or the myriad of other additives affected their digestion or health. Suspicious food additives included nerve tonics and invigorators, which were laced with cocaine, caffeine, chloral hydrates, and opium. Food preservatives targeted by the squad included boric acid or borax, a common additive in canned or tinned food. The study results warned consumers about these dangerous preservatives and additives. Several members of the squad had to quit before the study was completed because they were too sick to continue. Journalists, known as muckrakers, published investigative articles about the quality of everything from tinned meat and canned vegetables to patent medicines.

At the same time, the release of Upton Sinclair's novel *The Jungle* (1906)—with its vivid description of horrible conditions in meatpacking

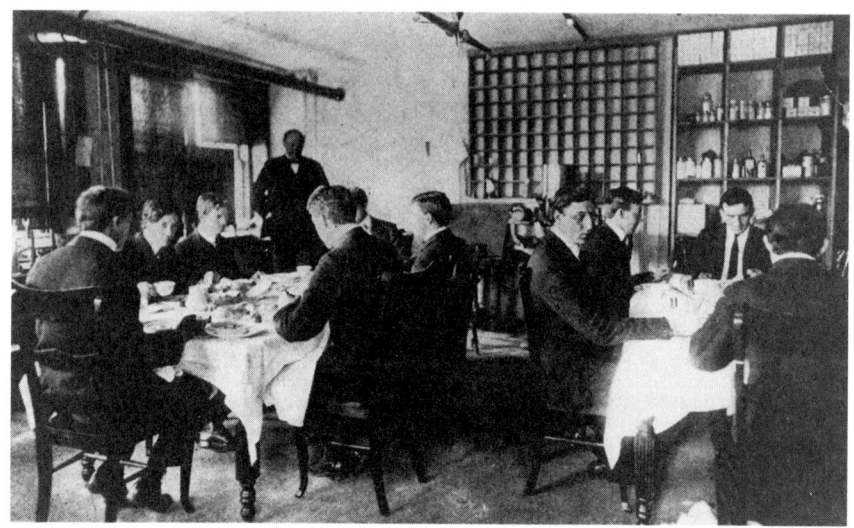

Dr. Harvey Washington Wiley and his volunteers, known as the "Poison Squad," turned themselves into human guinea pigs to study the effects of chemical preservatives in food during the early 1900s. [Photo courtesy of the FDA History Office]

plants—added to the nation's shock about the meatpacking industry. Average Americans angrily demanded more protection and better controls from the government over what went into food and drugs. President Theodore Roosevelt agreed, and signed the Pure Food and Drug Act, known as the Wiley Act, into law in 1906. The new legislation centered on product labeling and purity: no food or drug could be sold in any changed condition unless those changes were plainly stated on its label. The law prohibited any additives that would substitute for food, conceal damage, pose a health hazard, or constitute a filthy or decomposed substance. Based on the success of the 1906 legislation, Wiley accepted an invitation the following year to work with the French government and revise their food laws.

After almost 30 years at the Bureau of Chemistry, Wiley resigned in 1912. At that point, the agency turned its focus away from food additives and devoted more manpower to drug regulation, with an emphasis on patent medicines; it was renamed the Food and Drug Administration in 1930. By the 1930s, muckraking journalists were pushing Congress to update the 1906 Food and Drug Act and close its many loopholes. Food technology had changed rapidly and the number of possible ingredients going into foods and drugs had increased, making the old law grossly ineffective. New bills bounced back and forth between the House and Senate for several years, but Congress failed to pass any meaningful legislation.

It took a tragedy to break the stalemate. In 1937, over 100 people died from a single toxic medicine known as Elixir Sulfanilamide. Sulfanilamide, a tablet used to treat sore throats, was adapted to a liquid form by Massengill, a Tennessee drug company. The company's chief chemist and pharmacist discovered that the sulfanilamide powder easily dissolved in a liquid called diethylene glycol. The new medicine tasted like raspberries, and had a cheerful red color and a pleasant fragrance. Unfortunately, the liquid was a highly toxic variant of antifreeze. It was shipped all over the country during September and October of 1937. At that time, food and drug laws did not require safety studies on new drugs.

Without any premarket evaluation, the company's chemist failed to realize the danger until adults and children started taking the medicine. Complaints flooded the American Medical Association (AMA), which immediately gathered samples to isolate the toxic ingredient. The AMA also issued a warning through newspapers and the radio, but Americans continued drinking the elixir. The company sent telegrams to the salesmen, druggists, and doctors who purchased the elixir. The FDA also demanded that a second warning be publicized describing the risk.

FDA employees would eventually track down every single shipment, in some cases following the trail from drugstores to private homes in an attempt to recover all the elixir. There was no antidote or treatment, only a slow, painful death that began with nausea and vomiting and ended in convulsions, kidney failure, and death. When the episode was over, more than 100 people in 15 states had died, many of them children. The public was outraged, and their anger forced Congress to enact the 1938 Food, Drug, and Cosmetic Act. President Franklin Roosevelt signed it into law the next year.

UPDATED LEGISLATION

The 1938 law added cosmetics and medical devices to the list of items under FDA control, and required drugs and patent medicines be labeled with adequate directions for use. Most importantly, the law demanded presale approval of all new drugs, meaning a manufacturer had to prove that its drugs were safe before they could be sold. This corrected many abuses of quality standards. Still, problems remained. To answer continued complaints, the agency developed recipe standards for foods as well as for lists of ingredients included with products. Any food that deviated from a recipe had to be labeled as an "imitation."

In the early 1950s, a series of laws addressing pesticide residues and food and color additives gave the FDA greater power to regulate the growing list of chemical additives, and again put the responsibility on manufacturers to prove safety first. The FDA also challenged false nutritional claims in court. Each decade brought sensational cases, such as the aminotriazole-tainted cranberries in the 1950s and the vitamin fortification of foods and misleading health claims in the 1970s.

In 1973, the FDA ordered nutrition labeling for fortified foods with one or more added ingredients, but left labeling voluntary for all other food products. A decade later, in 1984, the pressure for standardized nutrition label information got a big push from the Center for Science in the Public Interest. The National Labeling and Education Act (NLEA) was passed in 1990. It required manufacturers of food products to put a uniform nutrition fact label on each package.

Current labels, by law, must include the amounts, per a specified serving size, of total fat, calories from fat, energy as calories, sodium, cholesterol, dietary fiber, total carbohydrate, protein, sugars, vitamins A and C, and the minerals iron and calcium. In addition, Percent Daily Values for these nutrient categories are given based on a diet of 2,000 calories per day. In 2006, the FDA added trans fat to the nutrition label requirements, and now requires food manufacturers to list trans fatty acids or trans fat if a food contains at least 0.5 grams of trans fat.

THE USDA AND NUTRITION

The government's role in accurate labeling, and in collecting and updating information on the composition of foods, has grown exponentially thanks to the USDA Human Nutrition Information Service (HNIS) and the Department of Health and Human Services National Center for Health Statistics. These two federal agencies conduct major national surveys, research nutrient requirements, and provide nutrition education to the American public in the form of dietary guidelines. The history of government attempts at public dietary guidance dates all the way back to W. O. Atwater's founding of the USDA Office of Experiment Stations in 1888. Atwater is best known for his elaborate tables listing the caloric values of many foods; much of his data is still in use today. Atwater also published *The Farmer's Bulletin,* filled with diets for American men that included recommended intake levels of protein, carbohydrates, and fat. Specific minerals and vitamins were not listed because they had not yet been discovered.

The next USDA publication appeared as a booklet aimed at improving the nutrition of young children. Titled *Food for Young Children* (1916), it was written by nutritionist Caroline Hunt. She divided foods into five distinct nutritional groups: milk and meat, cereals, vegetables and fruits, fats and fatty foods, and sugars and sugary foods. Hunt and Atwater then teamed up to publish a guide for the general public, *How to Select Foods* (1917). In 1933, the government developed and published extensive family food plans that listed 12 major food groups it thought necessary for good nutrition: milk; potatoes and sweet potatoes; dry beans, peas, and nuts; tomatoes and citrus fruits; leafy green and yellow vegetables; other vegetables and fruits; eggs; lean meat, poultry, and fish; flours and cereals; butter; other fats; and sugars.

In 1941, following the National Nutrition Conference for Defense, the Food and Nutrition Board of the National Academy of Sciences released the first set of Recommended Dietary Allowances (RDAs). President Franklin Roosevelt publicly supported the new RDAs as a way to keep Americans healthy, in part because Germany was at war with much of Europe. On December 7, 1941, the Japanese bombed Pearl Harbor, and Roosevelt declared war on Japan. Just days later, Germany, led by Adolf Hitler, declared war on the United States. Nutrition was serious business; the government needed healthy men to fight if the nation went to war.

Americans nervously watched the fighting in England and France and the food rationing it created. At the same time, the U.S. government continued to release food guides to improve health and nutrition. The USDA released the Basic Seven food guide in 1943 as part of its *National Wartime Nutrition Guide*; later, this guide became the foundation for the 1968 RDAs. Government officials created the wartime publication to help Americans cope with limited supplies and food rationing. By 1956, the economy had rebounded and food was plentiful; rationing was a thing of the past. The USDA shortened the twelve food groups into the Basic Four—milk, meat, fruits and vegetables, and grain products—and added a recommended number of servings for each food group.

Even though the USDA offered suggestions and guides over the years, the first official *Dietary Guidelines for Americans* was released in 1980 by the USDA and HHS. It continues to be revised every five years. In 2006, the familiar RDAs gained flexibility and were renamed Reference Daily Intakes (RDIs). RDIs are now listed on food labels, and simply suggest the daily amount of vitamins and minerals healthy adults should consume based on current nutritional information. They can be adjusted to take into account variables such as age, sex, and fitness levels.

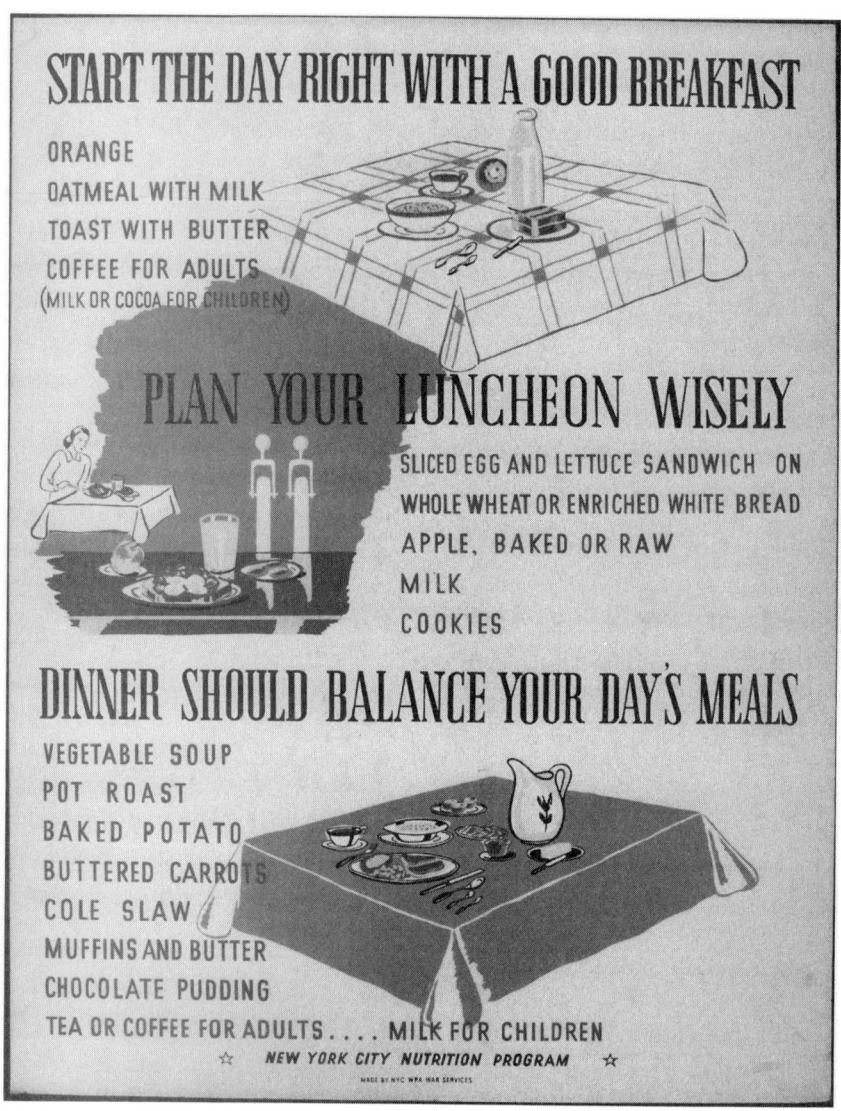

This 1941 New York City WPA War Services poster encouraged Americans to develop healthy eating habits. [Courtesy of Library of Congress]

Food Guide Pyramid

No mention of government nutrition education would be complete without inclusion of the Food Guide Pyramid. The Food Guide Pyramid is a visual reminder of a balanced and varied diet. The pyramid's predecessor, the Food Wheel was first released by the USDA in 1984 as part of a nutrition course developed in cooperation with the American National Red Cross. The Food Guide Pyramid was released in 1992 in an attempt to give the graphics a modern look. Several shapes were considered, but after a great deal of public input, the pyramid was chosen.

The newest adaptation of the now familiar shape is titled MyPyramid, and in 2005 it replaced the 1992 Food Guide Pyramid and associated materials. The new Pyramid incorporates recommendations from the 2005 Dietary Guidelines for Americans, released by the USDA in January 2005. The USDA calls the latest graphic a more personalized approach to healthy eating. The familiar shape shows a person climbing a set of steps, a reminder of the importance of daily activity. The different colors represent the variety of food groups available to consumers. The narrowing of each color band represents moderation; the wider base suggests foods to be eaten more frequently. The different widths of the food group bands indicate proportionality—how much food a person should choose from each group. Finally, the steps were designed to remind individuals that they can take small steps to improve their diet. The newest release includes calorie levels based on gender, age, and level of physical activity, and recognizes that each person's optimum nutrition is unique—that in the future, one size does not fit all.

SECTION TWO

Controversies and Issues Relating to Nutrition

CHAPTER 4

Food Irradiation: Past Its Shelf Life?

The room is quiet except for the hum of a conveyor belt. Thousands of potatoes, all boxed and stacked on the belt, glide through the vaulted room and are bathed in 100,000 rads of ionizing radiation from radioactive cobalt-60 rods lifted from deep pools of water. This is roughly the equivalent of 30 million X-rays. The whole operation takes just minutes as the potatoes complete their conveyor belt journey. Once they have been irradiated, the potatoes will not sprout eyes, and they may not spoil as quickly. They are irradiated so they can be shipped thousands of miles, and stored for weeks and months, before being sold and made into commercial foods such as French fries and mashed potatoes.

As the distance our food travels from field to table increases, scientists and consumers are asking with more urgency how we can keep our food supply safe. Recalls of meat, vegetables, and fruits are now commonplace. The largest recall to date of ground beef occurred in California in February 2008, when the U.S. Department of Agriculture (USDA) recalled over 143 million pounds of ground beef from a California slaughterhouse. The Centers for Disease Control and Prevention (CDC) estimate that every year, more than 76 million people become ill from something they have eaten, and of these, some 5,000 die from a variety of foodborne diseases.[1] Although food can be treated with irradiation to improve its safety, this decades-old idea still raises strong emotions, and—as with any controversial issue—there are two sides to the argument with two vastly different opinions.

IRRADIATION DEFINED

Food irradiation is a way to preserve food and extend its shelf life by exposing that food, either prepackaged or in bulk, to very high-energy, invisible light waves or radiation. Supporters compare the irradiation of food to the pasteurization of milk, using the phrase "cold pasteurization" to describe the process. Like pasteurization, irradiation kills a number of harmful bacteria, but not all, which means foods can be reinfected if not handled properly. Critics of irradiation argue that it is nothing like pasteurization. They challenge the food industry to instead reduce harmful bacteria by cleaning up the process of food handling itself. Critics fear that irradiation may do more harm than good to the very people it is designed to protect.

There are three basic types of energy used for irradiation: X-rays, electron beams, and gamma rays. The majority of irradiated meat is processed using electron beam or gamma ray technology. Gamma rays are produced by cobalt-60 or cesium-137—radioactive substances, called radioisotopes, that continuously emit dangerous rays when not submerged in water. A cobalt-based irradiator consists of a rack of radioactive rods, and requires a substantial amount of space to house the 15-foot-deep pool of water needed to absorb and neutralize the gamma rays when the rods are not in use. Conveyor belts carry the food around the radioactive rack so the rays can penetrate all sides. The rays can penetrate food to a greater depth than electron beams, so irradiation treatment times vary: fresh strawberries might take 5 minutes, whereas frozen meat would need up to 20 minutes of treatment time.[2] Like cobalt-60 irradiators, cesium-137 irradiators are stored in pools of water when not in use. They use fuel from decommissioned nuclear weapons and other radioactive waste. Cesium is water-soluble, making it very dangerous in the event of an accident, and it remains radioactive for hundreds of years, making it expensive to store.

Electron beam, or e-beam, irradiators lack penetrating power, but they do deliver faster and higher doses of radiation than gamma ray irradiators. They can only penetrate up to four inches, making them suitable for flat products such as hamburger patties. Food packaged in cartons is usually too thick to be processed with this method. The electron beams are not from radioactive sources, so they do not create radioactive waste; however, they do generate ionizing changes in foods. Ionizing radiation works by damaging the DNA of disease-causing bacteria such as *Salmonella* and *E. coli*; it either kills the microorganisms or genetically alters them so they can't reproduce. Whereas higher doses damage molecules in the food, lower doses damage only microorganisms and insects. Another positive aspect of e-beams is that the energy produced can be adjusted or turned off, making them safer for the environment and for workers.

The development of X-ray technology for irradiation is a blend of the other two techniques. X-rays penetrate like gamma rays, but are nonradioactive like electron beams. Produced by machines more powerful than those used in hospitals or dental offices, X-rays used in food irradiation penetrate well but have a slower processing speed. This means that larger volumes can be irradiated with X-ray systems, but that the process takes longer to accomplish.

Whichever method is used, food is irradiated at one of three dose levels—a dose being the amount of radiation absorbed by the food. The dose is based on the intensity of the radiation used and on the length of time it is applied. In the early days of the technology, doses were measured in rads—short for "radiation absorbed dose." However, the U.S. Food and Drug Administration (FDA) later switched from the rad to the gray (Gy), which is equal to 100 rads. A kilogray (kGy) is equal to 1000 Gy. To kill *Salmonella* bacteria, chicken receives from 1 to 10 kGy. For comparison, a single chest X-ray gives a dose of only half a milliGray—many million times less radiation than is delivered to the chicken.[3]

Over the years, the FDA has approved irradiation treatment for various types of food at low, medium, or high dose levels. A low dose is up to 1 kGy, and is applied to control insects in grains, stop potatoes from sprouting, control trichinae in pork, and delay decay in fruits and vegetables. Medium doses, from 1 to 10 kGy, are used to neutralize *Salmonella, E. coli, Campylobacter,* and *Shigella* in meat, poultry, and fish, as well as to delay the growth of mold on strawberries and other fruits. The highest doses, above 10 kGy, can kill microorganisms and insects in spices, and commercially sterilize foods to the same degree as canning. These highest doses are used for special hospital diets given to immune-compromised patients. Hospitals and other medical facilities routinely use radiation to sterilize equipment. This began in the mid-1960s, when a division of Johnson & Johnson sterilized sutures using radiation. Today, the United States has more than 40 licensed irradiation facilities, and most are used to sterilize medical and pharmaceutical supplies as well as other consumer products such as bandages, baby-bottle nipples, and cosmetic raw materials.

It is important to note that irradiation does not kill viruses, the bacteria that cause botulism, or the prions thought to cause mad cow disease (also known as bovine spongiform encephalopathy). It also does not eliminate the possibility of cross-contamination, especially of meat. Irradiated meat can still become contaminated if handled improperly, so consumers need to follow the same cooking and handling methods as with regular meat. For this reason, opponents question the benefit of

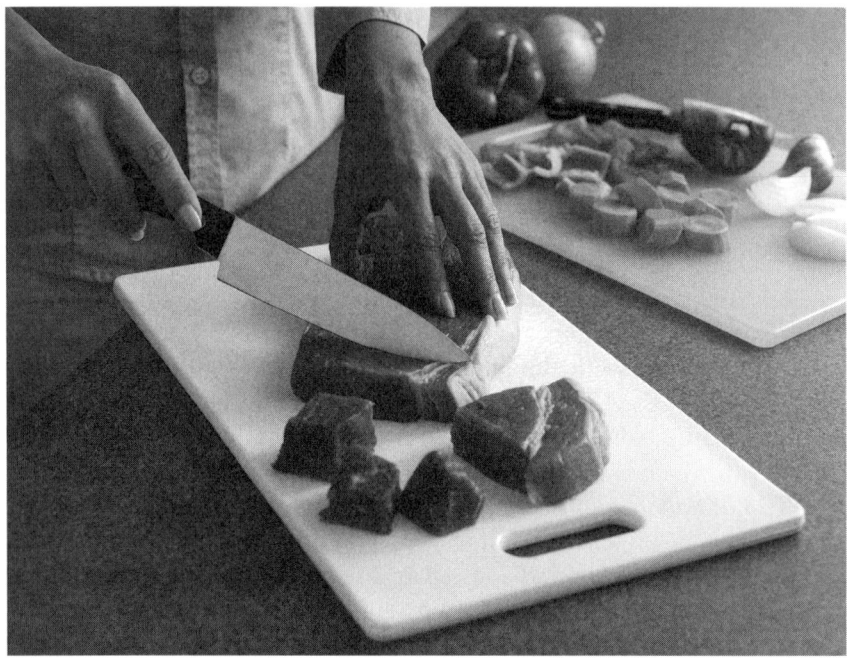

Irradiation of meat can kill harmful bacteria, but safe food handling and cooking methods must still be maintained to prevent foodborne illness. [Courtesy of the USDA Food Safety and Inspection Service]

food irradiation. They argue that no real need exists if people follow traditional food safety rules, and especially if the food industry significantly improves how food is handled during processing.

Early History

French physicist Antoine-Henri Becquerel was the first scientist to harness radiant energy or radiation. For his part in the discovery of the radioactivity of uranium salts, Becquerel shared the 1903 Nobel Prize in physics with Marie and Pierre Curie. Marie Curie was Becquerel's graduate student at the time, and was involved in an intensive study of radiation for her doctoral thesis. Curie was the first woman to win the Nobel Prize, and one of the few scientists to win it twice.

It was American biologist Samuel Prescott who linked radiation with food safety in 1904. A professor of biology at the Massachusetts Institute of Technology (MIT), Prescott initiated studies on the effect of gamma rays from radium on bacteria, and demonstrated that the rays could kill bacteria in food. However, the lack of suitable radiation sources and their high cost hindered his research. That same year, he founded the Boston Biochemical Laboratory so he could continue his work on the problems of bacteria in preserved food.

It was 50 years later that commercial irradiation of food finally kicked into high gear. On December 8, 1953, President Dwight Eisenhower stood before the United Nations General Assembly and gave his "Atoms for Peace" address. The Atoms for Peace program, spearheaded by the U.S. Atomic Energy Commission, aimed to use atomic energy for peaceful purposes. Eisenhower also formed the National Food Irradiation Program, which launched research projects on food irradiation sponsored by both the Atomic Energy Commission and the U.S. Army. The Army then conducted a series of experiments with fruits, vegetables, dairy products, fish, and meats, with an eye toward providing sterile foods that they could substitute for canned or frozen meals for soldiers, particularly in combat situations.

The nuclear age brought with it large sources of radiation materials, but consumers were afraid of anything suggesting nuclear exposure after seeing the effects of the explosions at Hiroshima and Nagasaki. Americans also connected the concept of radiation with nuclear power plants and medical X-rays, both caution-filled technologies that constantly guard against unnecessary exposure. To this day, discussion of food irradiation elicits a very emotional response from opponents of the technology, based on these same fears.

When U.S. consumers reacted negatively to the early introduction of gamma irradiation for treating food, American lawmakers realized they had to maintain tight control of this developing technology—especially because, up to that point, it had been completely funded by the government. In crafting the 1958 Food, Drug, and Cosmetic Act, Congress defined food irradiation as an additive rather than a process. This decision was intended to guarantee oversight and testing by the Food and Drug Administration (FDA) as manufacturers became involved in irradiation and rolled out new products. Ironically, early supporters considered irradiation a way to improve food safety without using chemical additives.

Defining irradiated foods as additives also ensured that those foods and their packaging would need FDA approval. Moreover, if animal products were involved, approval from the U.S. Department of Agriculture (USDA) was necessary as well. FDA regulations still require manufacturers seeking approval for irradiation products to file a food additive petition with either agency after gathering data to demonstrate safety. USDA regulations also mandate that workers be trained in the safe operation of irradiation equipment. Manufacturers who choose to irradiate meat or meat products need to comply with USDA Food Safety and Inspection Service (FSIS) and FDA requirements, as well as with regulations from the Nuclear Regulatory Commission, the Environmental Protection Agency, the Occupational Safety and Health Administration, the Department of Transportation, and state and local governments.

Even with oversight from so many government agencies, the question of safety testing remains a controversial issue and a battleground between supporters and opponents of irradiation technology. The 1958 act called on the government to set up safe conditions of use and parameters that irradiated food must meet. However, beginning in the 1960s, when the first petition for the treatment of food with radiation was submitted to the FDA, the agency failed to decide on test procedures to establish a reasonable certainty of no harm. Following decades of debate, the final statute did not come until April of 1986, and did not prescribe what safety tests should be performed, instead leaving that determination to the "discretion of scientists."[4]

In 1963, the FDA approved irradiation of wheat, flour, and canned bacon using cobalt-60 gamma rays, largely on the basis of early research by the U.S. Army. Other products quickly followed, including wheat and wheat products irradiated to control insect infestation. A few weeks later, the FDA again approved irradiation of canned bacon, this time using electron beam radiation at 45 to 56 kGy. The following year, the FDA amended the regulation to include irradiation of white potatoes to inhibit sprout development using cobalt-60 at 50 to 100 Gy.

LABELS AND PACKAGING

Other changes were made to the regulation, detailing radiation types and doses for a growing list of products, but it wasn't until 1965 that the USDA issued a regulation requiring the labeling of irradiated foods. This new regulation required that the phrase "Processed by ionizing radiation" appear on the labels. It was the first explicit government labeling requirement.[5] The regulations were amended several times, with the final statement, effective on March 2, 1967, remaining in place until April 18, 1986.[6] The labeling regulations required various statements, including "Treated with ionizing radiation" on retail packages of low-dose-treated foods; "Treated with ionizing radiation—do not irradiate again" on wholesale packages of bulk shipments of low-dose-treated foods; and "Processed by ionizing radiation" on foods treated with high-dose gamma ray, electron beam, and X-ray radiation. Manufacturers were allowed to replace the term "ionizing radiation' with "gamma-radiation," "electron radiation," or X-radiation" as appropriate.

All foods must be completely packaged before being irradiated, so several petitions for packaging materials were submitted for approval to the FDA beginning in 1965. The regulations were amended several more times as the agency worked to establish clear rules in a rapidly developing technology. However, the FDA continued to wrestle in particular with the issue of how to test irradiated foods for safety.

Historically, the FDA has used feeding studies to determine the safety of a food additive. By the spring of 1967, there was growing concern that petitions for irradiated foods were not meeting the agency's safety standards and were failing to win approval. That year, the FDA's Bureau of Science conducted a seminar for government scientists and administrators to improve the quality of petitions in the hope of increasing the petition approval rate. The report issued from that seminar by the associate director of the Bureau of Science addressed key questions, including, "What is the significance of radiation-induced mutations in microorganisms?"; "What is a sound basis for extrapolation of data from one product to another, from one species to another, or from one level of exposure to another?"; and "What is the significance of the destruction of vitamins?"[7]

Those questions were not immediately answered due to the growing concern over the quality of safety data. The situation came to a head in 1968, when the FDA rejected a petition for radiation-sterilized ham that relied on many of the same reports submitted in the original, successful petition for radiation-sterilized bacon in 1963. In a move that received little media attention, the agency revoked the regulations for high-dose gamma ray, electron beam, and X-ray radiation processing of canned bacon in October 1968. The FDA reported noticeable problems in animal studies that raised doubts about the safety of irradiated bacon, listing "significant adverse effects on reproduction in animals fed irradiated bacon, increased death rates in rats and reduced red blood cell counts in dogs and rats." The report added, "Indications were also present that animals on the irradiated diets may show a higher incidence in the development of cataracts and tumors than animals on control diets."[8]

However, even with these concerns about irradiated bacon, another decade passed before the FDA decided to revisit its policies on testing. In 1979, the agency established the Bureau of Foods Irradiated Food Committee (BFIFC) to make recommendations for establishing toxicological testing that would adequately assess the safety of irradiated foods. This time the first questions the committee tackled concerned what exactly should be tested, and what the difference was between an irradiated and an nonirradiated food. The committee focused on any products formed during the irradiation process, and eventually concluded that 10 percent of the products of the process were substances not normally present in non-irradiated food. The BFIFC used the term "unique radiolytic products" (URPs) to describe these substances introduced into food by irradiation.

The committee suggested that URPs would be formed in minute amounts if products were treated at doses below 1 kGy. Based on this assumption, the BFIFC concluded that this small quantity of URPs would be diluted in a large amount of food. They therefore waived the requirement for animal feeding tests, holding that the tests would not provide any significant findings and would be a waste of time and taxpayer dollars. Additionally, the BFIFC recommended that foods comprising no more than 0.01 percent of the daily diet, and irradiated at 50 kGy or less, be considered safe for human consumption without toxicological testing.[9]

When critics brought up the irradiated bacon study results, the agency responded that the numbers of animals examined in those studies was too small, and that the studies were of too poor a quality to have any statistical significance. The FDA agreed with the BFIFC conclusion, and ruled that adequate safety was demonstrated without the toxicological testing. The FDA adopted the BFIFC recommendations on March 27, 1981.[10] Later that year, the FDA's Bureau of Foods stepped in and gathered a second team of scientists, called the Irradiated Foods Task Group, to review all the available data and to put to rest any lingering safety concerns.

The goal of this task group was to compile and summarize any toxicology data available at the time, and to identify patterns and report any adverse findings. Their final report was in agreement with the BFIFC and the FDA that any toxicological testing of irradiated foods was too insensitive to accurately measure problems, given the low concentrations of URPs in irradiated foods. There was no discussion of potential problems associated with any cumulative effects. The task group determined that although toxicological data could be helpful in evaluating the safety of irradiated foods, it was not scientifically necessary. Instead, chemical formulas were created and used to predict the amounts of irradiated food a person might eat and what effect that food would have on overall human health.

At the same time, the FDA continued to approve irradiation requests. In 1983, approval was granted to use irradiation to kill insects and control microorganisms in a specific list of herbs, spices, and seasonings. In 1985, the FDA approved irradiation of pork to control trichinosis. In 1986, approval was given for irradiation to control insects and inhibit mold growth and ripening in a number of fruits, vegetables, and grains. In 1990, poultry was added to the list—although irradiation only reduces and does not eliminate all bacteria, so irradiated poultry still requires refrigeration. The FDA approved irradiation of red meat in 1997, with a dose of 4.5 kGy for uncooked, refrigerated meat and 7 kGy for frozen meat and meat products.

OPPONENTS

There is no question that food irradiation is an effective way to kill bacteria. However, opponents of the technology say it is not the best way to ensure the safety of America's food supply. Despite widespread support of irradiation from government, industry officials, and scientists, critics call food irradiation an untested experiment on American consumers. They argue that there is a lack of testing and an attempt by the government to disregard any tests showing adverse effects.

One of the most vocal opponents of food irradiation is the watchdog organization Public Citizen. This group was founded by consumer advocate Ralph Nader, and has been in operation since 1971. Public Citizen has charged the FDA with ignoring studies indicating that food irradiation may be dangerous, especially in light of the test results that caused the agency to revoke approval of irradiated canned bacon. The organization's chief fear concerns the unknown effects of eating irradiated food over time. They argue that irradiation creates toxic substances in the food. For example, critics point to a 1986 FDA statement identifying detectable quantities of hydrogen peroxide, organic peroxides, and hydroperoxides formed during irradiation of foods. These peroxides are the result of free radical chemical exchanges between oxygen and the radiolytic products from the carbohydrates, fats, oils, and water in food. The FDA considered the potential carcinogenicity of hydrogen peroxide created during irradiation, and concluded that there was no specific evidence that it would damage healthy cells before it was neutralized by natural enzymes or antioxidants in the food.

Public Citizen and other opponents also note that *Clostridium botulinum* spores may survive irradiation and produce botulinum toxin in food. Consumers would not notice the toxins, because irradiation prevents typical signs of spoilage. The FDA identified this as a legitimate concern in its April 1986 rules. The agency found that irradiation below 1 kGy will destroy only a few spoilage bacteria, and will not change the essential spoilage patterns of the food. In other words, the food will continue to rot even after it is irradiated, and that decay should alert consumers to the potential for other toxins.

Public Citizen and others have additionally suggested that irradiation may create potentially harmful radiation-resistant bacteria or viral mutants. Although the FDA admitted that mutants are produced during the irradiation of food, it labeled them "essentially the same as those that occur naturally."[11] Government scientists acknowledged that radiation may increase the frequency of mutations, and the FDA reported that this effect on the rate at which mutations occur is the only meaningful impact of irradiation on mutations. However, the FDA ruled that this was not a significant problem.

Other opponents of irradiation have claimed that the FDA has not addressed the destruction of vitamins and other important nutrients during radiation treatments. The Organic Consumers Association (OCA), a nonprofit public interest group, was formed in 1998 as part of a backlash against proposed changes to USDA organic food regulations. In addition to calling for a global moratorium on genetically modified foods, the association has been a vocal critic of irradiation. The OCA estimates that irradiated foods can lose up to 80 percent of important vitamins, including vitamins A, C, E, and B. They claim that different foods lose different vitamins, and that the loss increases with the radiation dose and with the storage time of each food. Over time, critics argue, this loss of vitamins and nutrients will hurt impoverished nations already dealing with inadequate nutrition. Supporters of irradiation say nutrient losses can be minimized by irradiating food in an oxygen-free environment or by irradiating food when it is cold or frozen.

Another strong anti-irradiation advocate is Food & Water Watch, a national environmental organization based in Vermont. This group suggests that the government is approaching the issue of foodborne illness from the wrong direction. They advocate an immediate cleanup in the current system of food production, especially in slaughterhouse facilities, factory farms, and large-scale vegetable and fruit production sites. They claim that irradiation only masks filthy conditions in massive livestock slaughterhouses and food processing plants. They also suggest that better testing of water used for washing fruits and vegetables could adequately combat bacteria. For example, the *E. coli* outbreak behind the California spinach recall of 2006—which killed one person and sickened hundreds more in 26 states—was ultimately thought to have derived from infected manure from a local cattle ranch.

Food & Water Watch warns that the cost of irradiating the U.S. food supply would dramatically raise food prices for consumers. They estimate that in order to irradiate the 8 billion pounds of hamburger Americans eat every year, the industry would have to build "80 multi-million dollar irradiation facilities."[12] When the costs of transportation and handling are added, Food & Water Watch calculates that consumers would see a jump of up to one dollar per pound in the price of ground beef, in contrast with the USDA estimate that the price per pound would increase by only a few cents.

In 2003, Public Citizen joined with the Center for Food Safety (CFS) to challenge FDA approval of irradiated meat. The CFS is a Washington-based food activism group established in 1997 by its sister organization, the International Center for Technology Assessment. Their stated purpose is to challenge harmful food production technologies with a goal of promoting sustainable alternatives. Their petition with Public Citizen called for existing approval of irradiated meat to be revoked in light of new toxicity studies, which, they charged, the FDA had failed to mention or consider in the 1997 approval of irradiated meat.

SUPPORTERS

The International Food Information Council (IFIC) is a key player on the other side of the debate over irradiated food. The IFIC was created to communicate science-based information on food safety and nutrition to government officials, educators, journalists, nutrition and health professionals, and others who work with consumers. The council is financed thanks to a number of companies in the food, beverage, and agricultural industries. The IFIC is based in Washington DC and focuses primarily on U.S. issues. However, according to its Web site, the IFIC recognizes the global nature of food and health issues, and therefore added "international" to its name. The organization does participate in an informal network with food information groups in Europe, Asia, Australia, Canada, Japan, New Zealand, and South Africa.

The International Irradiation Association (iiA) is another group focused on supporting the growth of food irradiation. The iiA was developed in 2003 to improve communication between irradiation industry members and special interest groups. Members include companies with an interest in every aspect of radiation technology, among them Johnson & Johnson, E-Beam Services, and China Biotech Corporation. The mission of iiA, according to its Web site, is to provide support to its members in advancing the use of irradiation technology around the world. The association also lobbies various government agencies. The Web site, which was launched in 2004, links members, offers updates on legislation, creates position papers on changes in the technology, and serves as a forum for member concerns.

The American Dietetic Association boasts more than 68,000 members. Calling itself the nation's largest organization of food and nutrition professionals, this group is also among the country's strongest supporters of food irradiation. The ADA position statement on food irradiation was released in 2000, and calls on association members, along with "government, food manufacturers, food commodity groups and qualified food and nutrition professionals," to "work together to educate consumers about this additional food safety tool and make this choice available in the marketplace."[13] As an advocate organization for the public on food and nutrition issues, the ADA strongly encourages its members to support the availability of irradiated foods, and has worked to make educational resources available to consumers on local, national, and international levels.

INTERNATIONAL ISSUES

Worldwide, about 50 countries have approved some 60 products to be irradiated. The United States, South Africa, the Netherlands, Thailand, and France are among the leaders in adopting irradiation technology.[14] Whereas food irradiation has been used for decades in the United States, the technology has been slow to find support in many parts of Europe, especially the United Kingdom. The British Food Standards Agency (FSA) was set up as an independent government department in 2000 to protect the public's health and consumer interests in relation to food. In 2007, they recommended no changes to their current permitted uses of irradiated food. There are seven categories of irradiated food permitted in the United Kingdom, including fruit, vegetables, cereals, bulbs and tubers, spices and condiments, fish and shellfish, and poultry. All items must be labeled "irradiated" or "treated with ionising radiation." Imported irradiated food is only allowed in the United Kingdom if it was treated in an authorized plant and accompanied by full documentation relating to that treatment. The United Kingdom will accept herbs or spices irradiated in non-EU countries, but only if the facilities are approved by the European Community.

From the beginning, European governments showed little interest in financing the research needed to advance radiation technology in their countries. In an early effort to move development forward, the International Atomic Energy Association (IAEA) established a Joint Expert Committee on Food Irradiation (JECFI) that joined with the United Nations Food and Agriculture Organization (FAO) as well as the World Health Organization (WHO). Beginning in 1964, this alphabet soup of organizations—the IAEA, FAO, and WHO—held a series of meetings to assess the quality and safety of irradiated foods. From those meetings came a series of reports, which concluded that all irradiated foods were safe to eat.

In 1997, the Joint FAO/IAEA/WHO Study Group on High Dose Irradiation released their final report, which stated, "food irradiated to any dose appropriate to achieve the intended technological objective is both safe to consume and nutritionally adequate." They added that "no upper dose limit need be imposed, and . . . irradiated foods are deemed wholesome throughout the technologically useful dose range from below 10 kGy to envisioned doses above 10 kGy."[15] The study group's overall objective was to standardize the EU member states' national laws on irradiation, and each member state was directed to implement legislation laid down in the group's directives. But doubts continued, and so did the debate.

As the irradiation industry sought a toe hold in Europe, several consumer groups strongly objected to food irradiation. The European Consumers' Organization (BEUC) suggested that, although products could be bacterially contaminated, the possibility of contamination was not an adequate justification for food irradiation and would never be a substitute for good hygiene practices. The BEUC also argued that the technology would give consumers the impression that products were safer, which in turn might lessen consumer vigilance in preventing cross-contamination. The European Community of Consumer Cooperatives (Euro Coop) argued that irradiation technology was an attempt to fix safety issues at the wrong end of the process. They suggested that it is possible to raise chickens in a *Salmonella*-free environment, thus placing the focus of food hygiene efforts on safety during production, storage, and manufacturing rather than at the last stage. They charged that irradiation would legitimize bad hygiene, and that an extended shelf life for irradiated foods would only benefit the producer, not the consumer. The British Medical Association stated that irradiation was not a response to technological need, and that it might encourage food producers to lower food safety standards. They called for irradiation to remain restricted to herbs, spices, and vegetable seasonings.

The United Kingdom took labeling regulations a step further in 2000, removing an exemption that allowed small amounts of irradiated foods in compound ingredients to remain unlabelled. The change means that any foods containing irradiated ingredients must now be labeled as such. Concerns were later heightened in Europe when research raised questions about substances known as 2-alkylcyclobutanones (ACBs)—byproducts created when fat in foods such as ground beef is irradiated. A 2003 study by Germany's Federal Research Centre for Nutrition suggested that 2-ABCs may promote colon cancer. This prompted the European Commission (EC) to place a moratorium on many irradiated foods. However, the EC will allow the approval of other irradiated foods in the future if all EU countries reach a consensus on which foods to allow. In the United States, the FDA had already approved the use of irradiation for a variety of foods, including meat, poultry, and eggs, before the German study was published in *Journal of Nutrition and Cancer* in December 2002. Although the German researchers warned against using the study results to discredit irradiation of meat, they also called for more scrutiny of 2-ACBs.

In direct contrast to the UK regulation, the United States requires labels on all irradiated foods except compound food products with irradiated ingredients. For example, potato soup made with irradiated potatoes, onions, and spices does not need to be labeled as irradiated, because the ingredients are not irradiated after they are combined. However, if irradiated potatoes are sold separately after they are irradiated, they must be labeled and carry the irradiation symbol. This parallels the differences in labeling requirements for genetically modified organisms (GMOs) in the United States and Europe. In Europe, foods containing any GMOs require labels, whereas in America, combined foods that use GMOs are not labeled. Americans who wish to avoid irradiated foods or genetically modified foods should select organically processed foods.

That may change, however, in light of a 2007 FDA proposal to modify the way irradiated food is labeled. The measure would allow manufacturers to petition the agency to forego a label entirely if the irradiation makes no material changes to the nutritional or functional properties of the food, or to use other terms for irradiation, such as cold pasteurization. Consumer and environmental groups have strongly protested the changes, whereas advocates of irradiation say this may jump-start the technology and improve consumer acceptance of irradiated products. The proposed rule change would only apply to FDA-regulated foods; the USDA would have to enact a similar regulation to change labeling requirements for meat, poultry, and other USDA products. The FDA continues to review the proposal with no stated timetable for a final decision.

THE FUTURE OF IRRADIATION

According to supporters of food irradiation technology, the most important reason to continue development is to make the nation's food supply safe. Other factors that support development include improved living standards for people around the world, and an end to food shortages for a growing world population. The technology was first developed as a way to improve food logistics for the U.S. Army, especially in combat situations. However, in 1970, the Department of the Army notified Congress that it would terminate its support of the Food Irradiation Program by the end of that year. Congress insisted that the Army reconsider, but to date the military has not integrated food irradiation in any measurable way into food preparation for U.S. troops.

Another important expectation was that food irradiation would assist the nuclear energy industry in better utilizing radioactive waste products, which would improve the economics of nuclear power use. Following the accident at the Three Mile Island nuclear power plant in Pennsylvania on March 28, 1979, and the meltdown at the Chernobyl nuclear power plant in what was then the Ukrainian republic of the Soviet Union on April 26, 1986, the use of nuclear energy has leveled off, and along with it the pressure to handle radioactive waste products.

Most importantly, supporters of food irradiation say it is a vital additional tool to keeping U.S. food safe. Opponents argue that food safety would be better served if people washed their hands and cooked their food carefully, that irradiation will not make food safe if it is not handled properly, and that it does not eliminate a very deadly and incurable food-related illness, mad cow disease (bovine spongiform encephalopathy).

Overall, both sides do agree that food irradiation supports the global trend of centralized mass production and distribution of foods worldwide—a trend that raises the price tag for individual consumers as oil prices climb and global warming increases. Prolonged shelf life means foods can be transported over greater distances. This brings food to isolated or impoverished areas, but also increases fuel consumption and pollution. Critics of irradiation argue that consumers, already facing rising food prices, would feel a bigger financial pinch if additional, expensive irradiation facilities were constructed.

The use of irradiation is largely unacceptable to European consumers. Americans, on the other hand, have shown some reluctance to purchase irradiated food when it is labeled as such, but otherwise have adopted a "don't ask, don't tell" attitude. Are irradiated foods safe to eat or a dangerous experiment using American consumers? After more than 50 years, it still depends on who you ask.

CHAPTER 5

Genetically Modified Food: Are We Playing God?

Imagine a world where nutrition and food are the best they can be, and where plants fight off insects, viruses, and weeds. Now imagine plants that grow to two or three times their original size and provide crop yields so abundant that there are no hungry people. Supporters of genetically modified (GM) foods believe this vision is the future.

On the other side of the argument is a world where a handful of giant corporations control the seed and food supply, and where all crops are doused with pesticides even though the plants contain those very poisons. In this scenario, pesticide-resistant weeds force farmers to use more and more toxic methods. This is a world where genes from the new plants mix with those of wild species and change crops in uncontrollable ways, where genetically modified foods create unexpected allergies or incurable diseases. Opponents of genetic engineering are convinced that such a world is an imminent danger.

The changes biotech scientists and researchers envision for plants, such as making them more nutritious or tolerant of droughts, would provide important advantages around the globe—especially in third world areas where farming is difficult and people face malnutrition and starvation. However, these benefits have yet to materialize. Instead, other changes have been made to plants strictly for the profits of the biotech corporations and the food processing industry, such as delayed ripening, extended shelf lives, and altered tastes and textures. These changes come from the same chemical companies that brought major environmental problems in the last half of the twentieth century. Critics fear that the corporations that doused us with DDT and poisoned the air and water are now allowed to change the very essence of our foods without major checks and balances in place.

Who protects the average consumer in the world of GM foods? What will biotechnology do to the environment and our health? Do GM foods really differ in meaningful ways from their traditional counterparts? To answer these questions, it's important to understand the basics of GM foods, to define the relevant terminology, and to profile supporters and opponents.

GENETIC MODIFICATION AND GENETIC ENGINEERING DEFINED

Genetically modified (GM) foods derive from genetically modified organisms (GMOs)—plants created for human or animal consumption using biotechnology instead of conventional plant breeding. The term most commonly used in the United States to describe the technology is genetic engineering (GE). Scientists and researchers describe the modified DNA produced in the process as recombinant DNA (rDNA). In Europe, genetic engineering is generally referred to as genetic modification, mainly because this term translates easily among different languages. The foods produced from genetic engineering are also called biotech foods, gene foods, bioengineered foods, gene-altered foods, transgenic foods, and, among the harshest critics of the technology, Frankenfoods.

Techniques for isolating and altering genes were first developed by American geneticists during the early 1970s. In 1982, researchers succeeded in transferring genes between plant species. In conventional plant breeding, seeds and plants can be improved, but not chemically altered. In a GM food, DNA changes occur thanks to scientists who

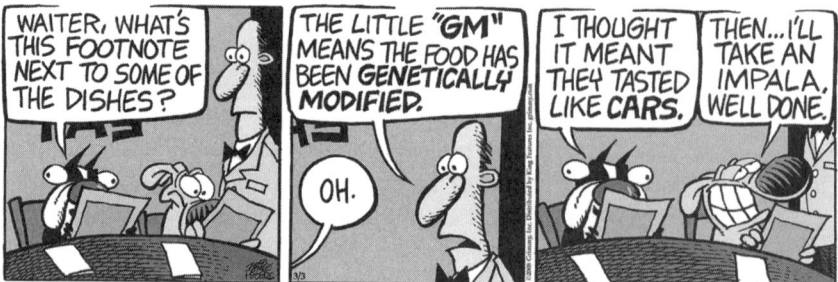

Comic strips like *Mother Goose and Grimm* have poked fun at the public's lack of understanding of genetically modified foods. [*Mother Goose & Grimm*— (new) © Grimmy, Inc., King Features Syndicate]

introduce specific traits into a plant by inserting one or more new genes into its genetic code. Unlike plants produced through conventional breeding, GM plants are given genes from vastly different organisms. To some, this is playing God; to others, it is science at its best. Although neither sinner nor savior, genetically modified organisms are at the epicenter of this ongoing debate.

Scientists have mixed the genes of animals and vegetables as well as those of vegetables and bacteria. The most widely used gene transfer is the introduction of a "Bt" gene into corn, cotton, or soy. Bt, or *Bacillus thuringiensis*—a naturally occurring bacterium—produces proteins that poison insect larvae. The Bt bacterium is related to the common bacterium responsible for food poisoning, and is also a close relative of the organism that causes anthrax. Surprisingly, Bt toxin has been used for years by organic growers, who spray it on plants to kill pests. The toxin breaks down rapidly after killing the pests, and there is no evidence of health problems for people eating food sprayed properly with it. When the Bt toxin genes are inserted into corn, the plants generate their own pesticides, allowing them to kill insects such as the corn borer. The long-term effects of eating Bt corn have not been studied to date.

ADVANTAGES AND DISADVANTAGES

Supporters of genetically modified foods say they offer several clear advantages, including pest resistance for crops, herbicide tolerance, disease resistance, and a better ability to withstand difficult growing conditions. The potential for improved nutrition, or for the development of new pharmaceuticals in foods such as tomatoes and potatoes, are expected to improve living conditions around the world.

Corporations such as Monsanto consider GM foods, especially Monsanto's Bt corn, a great success in protecting the environment by eliminating the overuse of chemical pesticides and herbicides. Thanks to the transfer of the Bt insect toxin genes, the plants do the work of the pesticides by easily killing the insects that feed on them. In addition to the Bt gene transfer, several crops (including Bt corn) have been genetically modified for resistance to weed-killing herbicide sprays. According to biotech companies, their statistics show that farmers who plant herbicide-tolerant plants reduce the amount of herbicide chemicals they spray on their crops. One prime example is the Monsanto strain of soybeans genetically modified to withstand the company's herbicide, Roundup. According to Monsanto, farmers who plant their soybeans use fewer applications of Roundup, thereby reducing costs and limiting dangerous chemical runoff.

Biotech companies also promote the eventual development of GM foods containing added vitamins and minerals, which they suggest will one day eliminate malnutrition around the world. Given these possibilities, corporate officials have little patience for critics, who they characterize as overzealous environmentalists with no scientific evidence to back up their charges.

The critics of GM foods are equally adamant about their concerns, which fall into three main categories: environmental hazards, human health risks, and economic effects. Critics worry about unintended harm to other plants, insects, and animals when GM crops spread through natural pollination, are carried away on the wind, and fertilize other plants. Scientists call this phenomenon gene flow. It occurs when the plants fertilized by stray crop pollen reproduce, and their offspring take on the herbicide- and pest-resistant characteristics of the GM crops. Some critics of genetic engineering believe that genes introduced to GM plants could spread uncontrollably or create unstoppable superweeds. Gene flow would force farmers to use stronger herbicides or risk losing their crops. Biotech corporations have suggested that farmers should combat gene flow by planting non-GM crops around the GM fields, creating a buffer zone.

Critics also predict that just as antibiotics have been overused, creating more antibiotic-resistant diseases, the overuse of pesticides on U.S. farms will mean chemical after chemical will become less effective—allowing superpests and superweeds to flourish. The Union of Concerned Scientists says there are signs that the most popular Bt crops will lose their effectiveness as weeds become resistant.[1] Scientists also expect those plants to fall victim to Bt-resistant pests.

Another environmental fear is that GM crops with pest-killing genes will destroy helpful insects. Opponents of GM foods say the monarch butterfly symbolizes this risk. In the spring of 1999, a laboratory study published in *Nature* indicated that pollen from Bt corn could kill the larvae of monarch butterflies.[2] At the time, Bt corn varieties had been planted on 20 million acres across the United States, including areas directly in the migratory path of the butterflies. Earlier tests on Bt crops by the Environmental Protection Agency (EPA) failed to consider the crops' potential effects on monarch butterflies, or on other moths or butterflies not damaging to crops. They only tested the Bt toxin's ability to kill the larvae of pests such as the corn borer.

Following the study's release, a storm of protests forced the U.S. Department of Agriculture (USDA) to review just how real the threat was to the monarch population. The results of the USDA's 2001 study showed that only one Bt corn variety had high enough levels of Bt toxin to easily

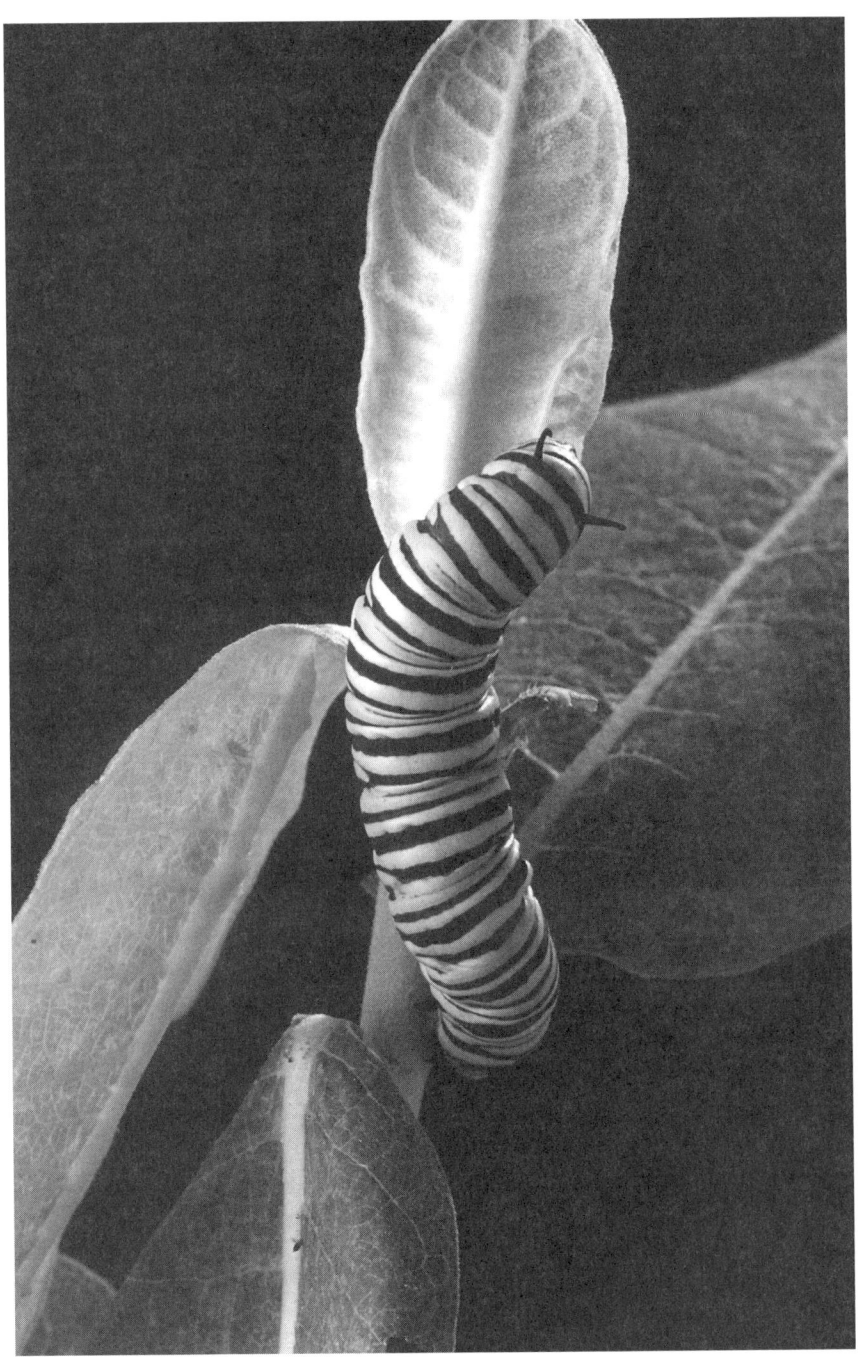

This monarch butterfly caterpillar symbolizes what environmentalists call the danger genetic engineering represents to useful insects when they feed on GM crops that contain pesticides. [Courtesy of the USDA Agricultural Research Service]

kill the monarch larvae. Luckily, that seed did not sell well and was not widely planted. But the crisis demonstrated a lack of government vigilance, and bolstered critics' claims that many insects, as well as animals higher up in the food chain, were at risk from GM crops. The 2001 USDA study did not address whether GM crops had the potential to cause future abnormalities, such as delayed development, impaired reproduction, altered growth, or shortened life spans.

The monarch butterfly was again center stage in the debate over GM foods in November 2007, when environmental officials with the European Union (EU) announced study results showing that two varieties of GM corn harmed butterfly species, specifically the monarch. In a statement, EU environment commissioner Stavros Dimas called the "potential damage on the environment irreversible," and said the level of risk generated by cultivation was unacceptable.[3]

Farmers and environmentalists opposed to GM plants also argue that altered seeds threaten biodiversity. Farmers have saved their seeds through hundreds and thousands of seasons, using each generation of seeds to improve properties such as resistance to pests, drought, wind, and changing weather. But the use of GM seeds, controlled by a few large biotech corporations, could eliminate many varieties of plants. Modern consumers may not realize that only one percent of vegetable varieties grown a century ago are still available for purchase today. If, or when, a crop is attacked by a new disease, as occurred with U.S. corn in 1970, today's researchers must look to a rapidly shrinking pool of heirloom seeds for solutions. Critics worry that someday those seeds simply won't exist if GM crops continue to cross-pollinate conventional fields.

Cross-pollination from GM crops has also been an important legal issue. Monsanto and other companies have sued farmers for patent infringement; Monsanto claims that the farmers obtained their GM seeds without paying royalties to the company. The farmers argued that the crops were the result of cross-pollination they could not control. Monsanto has won the majority of their patent infringement claims. The company has also successfully sued farmers who saved and planted seeds from those cross-pollinated fields. One suit against a Canadian farmer attracted considerable media attention. In that case the farmer had not purchased Roundup Ready Canola, but his fields became contaminated through cross-pollination. He then saved and replanted until his seeds contained a majority of the patented canola. Although the farmers have not been very successful in defending themselves, they continue to fight in the courts.

Opponents of GM foods fear that there are unstudied and potentially devastating health risks for humans who eat the foods, as well. Changing the fundamental DNA of a food could cause new diseases or health problems. At a minimum, critics argue, these untested genetic combinations could create proteins that trigger severe allergic reactions. One example that critics cite involved deaths from L-tryptophan, an amino acid pill that killed 38 people and sickened thousands in 1989. The Japanese manufacturer of the pill used genetically engineered bacteria in its production, and, although it is not clear how the toxins developed in the drug, opponents of genetic engineering suspect the bacteria was a factor. Ultimately, no definite cause was pinpointed, but scientists agreed that some people were genetically more likely to react fatally to the amino acid in its pure form. L-tryptophan was banned, and opponents of genetic engineering continue to raise questions about the role GM bacteria played in the tragedy.

Critics of GM foods say their greatest fear is the potential for such unknown human health consequences. They maintain that none of the genetically modified food crops currently on the market have been put through significant scientific studies or controlled testing to determine their overall effects on humans. The testing done to date, they argue, has been performed by the same companies that research, develop, and sell GM plants. Critics want the government to test GM crops using trials similar to those applied to new food additives.

Finally, critics of GM foods concerned with their effects on humans warn that the food supply could quickly be contaminated by allergens unexpectedly created in GM crops, as happened with StarLink corn contamination. In April 1997, the biotech firm Aventis Crop Science applied to the EPA for a license to sell StarLink, a genetically engineered Bt corn. However, introduction of the Bt gene in StarLink produced a protein, called Cry9C, not present in other Bt corn crops. Scientists noticed that this particular protein did not digest well in people and did not break down in heat, two major characteristics common when food proteins trigger allergic reactions.

Based on this information, the EPA rejected StarLink for human consumption, but granted a split registration that allowed it to be used for animal feed. StarLink was also not licensed for export. In September of 2000, StarLink was detected in Taco Bell taco shells, and the parent company, Kraft Foods, immediately issued a voluntary recall. In the months that followed, StarLink was discovered in more and more yellow corn products in the United States and in other countries.

To critics of GM foods, this episode raised serious questions about the U.S. government's ability to keep such foods separate from conventional foods. Before the StarLink incident was over, American companies were forced to recall over 300 contaminated food products in 2000 and 2001.

The incident heightened fears among European consumers. Corn exports from the United States to Europe were halted, and companies were forced to buy back contaminated corn. In the United States, farmers filed class-action suits in Nebraska, Iowa, and Illinois to recoup big losses that had resulted when their corn was contaminated or commingled with StarLink. Aventis eventually reached an agreement in 17 states to compensate farmers for their losses.

Surprisingly, StarLink represented only one percent of the total U.S. corn crop in 2000. However, when it accidentally mixed with other corn varieties, it may have contaminated up to 50 percent of the year's corn harvest. There were still more costs for Aventis. Following the discovery of StarLink contamination in foods, over two dozen people reported severe allergic reactions and filed a class-action suit. The FDA and the Centers for Disease Control and Prevention (CDC) tested blood samples from a majority of those people, and, although it did appear that the claimants suffered severe allergic reactions to something, the CDC ruled that StarLink was not responsible.

Aventis petitioned the EPA to allow the temporary approval of StarLink for human consumption based on this new data. But the EPA rejected the company's petition, and ruled that StarLink still posed a moderate allergy risk. The FDA then ordered mandatory testing of food for traces of StarLink. Testing continued for six years until the EPA and FDA placed a notice in the October 17, 2007, *Federal Register,* announcing that the level of risk from StarLink was low enough to end testing. Aventis reached a $9 million settlement of the class action lawsuit in 2002. Although company officials denied any liability for the claims, they called the settlement the best way to move forward. Aventis also voluntarily withdrew from its regulatory approval to sell StarLink corn in the United States, finally ending this costly episode.

Cost is a third key area of argument used by critics of GM foods, who argue that the foods are priced no more cheaply than their conventional counterparts and fail to benefit consumers nutritionally. Proponents of GM foods talk of future products, but it is true that bioengineered crops, at this time, modify the production characteristics of plants, not their health benefits. Biotech corporations reportedly have low-calorie and vitamin-enhanced products in the planning stages, but few have reached the marketplace. Another economic downside of GM foods, according to critics, is that patents are placed on GM seeds and prices go up, meaning small farmers may not be able to afford the engineered seeds. Because growers are not allowed to save GM seeds from year to year, if their conventional seeds are altered by the GM plants, small farmers may be left with nothing to grow. Critics say that, one way or another, small farmers will ultimately be squeezed out, leaving giant biotech companies in control of the world's seed and food supply.

HISTORY

Genetically modified crops were first commercially sold in 1995 in the United States. Ten years later, in 2005, a total of 21 countries reported planting GM crops, including the United States, Argentina, Brazil, China, India, South Africa, Canada, and Mexico.[4] The first genetically engineered food marketed anywhere in the world was America's FlavrSavr tomato. For years, growers had unsuccessfully tried to adapt the tomato, using conventional means, to meet the needs of a rapidly expanding U.S. market. Breeders carefully selected varieties with tougher skins, or ones that ripened slowly, to produce a tomato for shipping anywhere at any time of the year. Next, growers harvested green, hard tomatoes, and introduced ethylene into the process. Ethylene, commonly used as an anesthetic, became popular as a quick spray to ripen tomatoes long after they were picked.

In the late 1980s, Calgene, a biotech start-up company in California, discovered the enzyme that controlled the rotting process in tomatoes, and reversed its DNA sequence. The resulting "FlavrSavr" tomato turned red on the vine, but was firm enough to be shipped across the country before it turned to mush. Calgene was not legally required to perform tests or even to notify the government of its marketing plans. But, in early 1993, public worries about food safety pushed Calgene officials to ask the FDA for a ruling on the safety of their new, biologically altered tomato. Opponents of GM foods had already publicly ridiculed another company for inserting a fish gene from the Arctic flounder into a tomato to give it resistance to frost damage. Calgene officials hoped a positive FDA ruling on the FlavrSavr tomato might ease consumer concerns.

Following numerous submissions and hearings, the FDA gave its approval in May 1994, calling the FlavrSavr tomato "substantially equivalent" to its predecessors. This early decision had lasting ramifications, and opened the door for companies to introduce GM foods without premarket testing for safety or labels. FlavrSavr tomatoes, however, were clearly labeled as "genetically modified," and sold along with information pamphlets. Surprisingly, overall production of the tomatoes was hurt by unexpected problems, damage during shipping, and low tomato prices, rather than by the tomato's GM status.

The final blow to Calgene and the FlavrSavr tomato came in the form of a copyright infringement lawsuit filed against Calgene by Monsanto in 1995.

The embattled Calgene agreed to sell over 50 percent of its stock to Monsanto as part of the settlement. In 1997, Monsanto bought the rest of the company, along with the patents for the tomato, genetically modified cotton, and canola. Less than three years after its introduction, the FlavrSavr tomato disappeared.

Research continued on new varieties of GM tomatoes, but as of 2006, genetically engineered tomatoes were no longer grown anywhere in the world. Monsanto reported similar problems with its genetically engineered wheat. The company reversed plans to sell the wheat after conducting test fields in 2003. They cited a lack of buyers for GM wheat as the main reason, especially in Europe, where countries refused to sell GM products and demanded strict labeling. U.S. biotech companies learned great lessons from the introduction of the FlavrSavr tomato when it became very clear that shoppers here and in Europe would steer clear of GM-labeled foods. Although the FlavrSavr tomato was not a commercial success, it opened the door for future development. More importantly, it defined the need for careful marketing of foods by companies such as Monsanto, and provided a sneak preview of the U. S. government's response to GM foods.

GOVERNMENT'S ROLE

In the United States, three agencies have jurisdiction over genetically modified organisms (GMOs). They comprise the U.S. Department of Agriculture (USDA), the Food and Drug Administration (FDA), and the Environmental Protection Agency (EPA). Overall, the FDA has the bulk of the responsibilities for GMOs, because it is responsible for the safety and nutrition of food and food additives. In 1986, the Reagan administration formally published the "Coordinated Framework for Regulation of Biotechnology" that set up how the three agencies would divide their responsibilities. This trio was given the task of adapting existing statutes to govern the new science, based on the belief that it was similar to earlier reproductive technologies. Since 1986, the FDA has continually ruled that existing laws are adequate for regulating any new GM foods.

The most striking aspect of the system is that it remains voluntary. The FDA does not require safety reviews on GM foods, and only requires labeling if the composition of a GM food is radically different from that of its conventional counterpart. If a company voluntarily decides to submit a GM plant for evaluation, the end result is usually a statement from the FDA finding the engineered crop substantially equivalent to its nonengineered version. In other words, FDA policy begins with the premise that plants developed through biotechnology are not inherently unsafe or different in any significant way. They are evaluated on their physical characteristics rather than on how they were created. If it looks like a tomato, smells like a tomato, and tastes like a tomato, it must be a tomato, even if it contains genes from fish or bacteria.

The EPA has the strongest regulations of the three agencies, but plays a much smaller role in the regulation of biotechnology. The agency oversees the manufacture, sale, and use of plant pesticides and other toxic substances as well as beneficial insects and other living organisms. However, only two classes of GM plants fall under the EPA's control: plants containing Bt toxins with resistance to certain insects, and GM plants with a resistance to viruses.

The third agency, the USDA, oversees plants and plant pests and controls the testing of GM crops in order to protect U.S. crops from pests. If agricultural corporations can demonstrate to the USDA that their GM crop is not a pest, they are free to plant and sell the crop on U.S. farmland. A smaller agency within the USDA, the Animal and Plant Health Inspection Service (APHIS), also oversees the safety of GM organisms and their overall impact on U.S. agriculture. The service focuses on new GM plants, and evaluates potential problems with pests or weed escapes that could damage American agriculture.

Although several guidelines influence field testing of genetically modified plants, the USDA rarely rejects new GM plants. Between the years 1987 and 2005, APHIS approved more than 10,000 field test requests out of the 11,000 they received.[5] Field test approval leaves deregulation as the only real hurdle facing biotech companies before they can market a new GM food in the United States. After they gather several years of data from regulated field trials, developers go back to APHIS and petition for deregulation. If the petition is accepted—and the vast majority are—then the GM product is treated as equivalent to the conventionally grown product, and is sold to consumers without a label or any mention of genetic changes.

The FDA released a series of policy statements in 1992, including "Foods Derived from New Plant Varieties." This landmark statement said GM foods were presumed generally recognized as safe (GRAS) and marketable as such. It's important to remember that the FDA deals with food safety after a product is on the shelves. The agency first created and applied the idea of substantial equivalence in the case of the FlavrSavr tomato. The GRAS designation of GM foods cemented the policy that when the nutritional content of a GM food appears the same as its conventional version, the FDA will not require any testing or special labeling. As recently as 2006, the FDA published new policies calling for voluntary consultation with GM companies in the early stages of development.

According to FDA officials, early contact should successfully limit the accidental entry of new allergens or toxins into the U.S. food supply. The FDA also ruled that non-GM foods cannot be labeled as GM-free unless they carry a disclaimer stating that the label does not imply that GM foods are of a lesser quality.

Labeling

The argument against labeling genetically modified food is largely economic. Basically, those who favor GM foods take a strong stand against labeling, calling it cost-prohibitive, unnecessary, misleading, and inefficient. In the United States, GM plants are routinely harvested and mixed with conventional crops. Advocates of GM foods say the cost to consumers of segregating bioengineered foods from conventional foods would raise food prices but provide no other real benefits.

Opponents of GM foods already distrust such foods. They describe a complete lack of studies to support the industry's position, and argue that without scientific reassurance that GM foods are safe to eat, labels are vital for consumers who want to avoid the foods. Critics also point to legislation that exists outside the United States. They say it is in America's best interest to have internationally clear standards and labels rather than the current U.S. policy, which creates a distinct economic disadvantage for our farmers due to large export losses. Critics predict that labels are inevitable if the United States hopes to maintain important European export markets.

There is also speculation among consumer advocates that manufacturers of GM foods wish to avoid the greater cost of liability that labels would bring. U.S. insurance industry officials report that underwriters would charge more for policies for biotech companies if labels were mandatory in this country. In Latin America, insurers exclude GM crops from basic insurance policies, and charge a special premium to cover them. In the United States, the absence of labels eliminates liability for corporations by making it difficult for individuals to prove exposure to GM foods, or to identify, trace, or verify problems related to their consumption.

Legal Challenges

The StarLink case is one of the very few successful court challenges to genetically modified foods. However, the limited record of success did not stop consumer advocates from taking the FDA to court again. In 1998, a small group of American scientists, environmentalists, consumer advocates, and religious leaders with serious concerns about GM foods decided to challenge government policy. The Alliance for Bio-Integrity v. Shalala, et al., was filed in U.S. District Court in Washington DC. The Alliance sued the FDA for failing to require safety testing and labeling of GM foods, and charged that the government's policy endangered public health and violated the religious freedom of individuals who wished to avoid chemically altered foods. The group sought to raise public awareness of the FDA policy that does not require labeling or premarket approval of gene-altered foods. They argued that the rule leaves American consumers with no way of knowing what GMOs are on the market. In fact, the market is filled with GM foods. The Center for Food Safety (CFS) reported as of 2007 that an estimated 75 percent of processed foods on U.S. supermarket shelves now contain genetically engineered ingredients.[6] The CFS was started in the early 1990s to pressure the government to test the health and environmental consequences of biotech foods.

The 1998 legal challenge did shed some light on the FDA support of GMOs. During the trial, internal FDA documents and memos revealed that the agency's own scientists had expressed concerns about the safety of genetically altered foods, and that these concerns were ignored and suppressed. In her 2000 ruling, Superior Court Judge Colleen Kollar-Kotelly acknowledged that government files contained statements from FDA scientists about possible unique health risks from GM foods. However, the judge held that the agency's politically appointed administrators were within their legal rights to set policy contrary to the scientific opinions of their staff. The judge recognized several key points for the plaintiffs, but she ultimately found that the FDA was within its rights.

To win, the plaintiffs needed to demonstrate that the FDA had abused its discretion and had acted arbitrarily in assuming that GM foods were generally recognized as safe (GRAS). The judge ruled that there was some rational basis for the FDA's presumption of GRAS, and that the policy could be upheld. On the other hand, she called the FDA policy on GM foods essentially one of inaction that did not follow the advice and warnings of the FDA scientific staff about the foods. She also recognized that there continued to be significant disagreement among scientific experts about the safety of GM foods, a minor victory for the plaintiffs.[7]

European Response to GM Foods

Fear of genetically engineered food has flourished in Europe for decades, and has effectively stopped efforts by American biotech corporations to promote genetically modified crops in countries outside the United States. Despite scientific and industry reassurance that GM foods are safe for human consumption, and a ruling by the World Trade Organization (WTO) against import bans in the European Union, genetic engineering technology continues to be rejected by an overwhelming majority of Europeans. Internationally, some 35 countries have restrictions on GM foods, ranging from mandatory labeling to outright bans.[8] In comparison to their international counterparts, Americans seem unconcerned with the extent of GM foods in the U.S. marketplace.

Faced with overwhelming opposition to GM foods and a growing concern about a weak regulatory process, the European Commission—the executive body of the European Union—failed to approve any applications for the cultivation of genetically modified crops from 1998 to 2004. The United States criticized this unofficial ban, calling it a political roadblock with no scientific basis. In May 2003, the United States, Canada, and Argentina filed a complaint with the WTO to force the European Union to allow imports of GM foods.

The WTO was created in 1995 to oversee free trade around the globe. The Geneva-based group sets rules aimed at removing barriers to the import and export of products between nations and trading countries, and it mediates trade disputes between member nations. The WTO has the power to fine countries that ignore its rulings. The WTO ruled in 2006 that the European Union's unofficial ban on GM foods contradicted its rules, but problems continued as member states found ways to adopt their own bans.

By 2003, EU officials proposed a complex system requiring labeling of any food produced from a GM organism along with stringent traceability requirements throughout the food system. They demanded that GM products be separated from conventional products, and the separation documented. EU officials called their new requirements for traceability and labeling an important step in rebuilding consumer confidence in the EU food safety regulatory system and in GM foods in general. Slowly, European countries began in 2004 and 2005 to allow GM seeds into the EU Common Catalog. A seed cannot be sold or exchanged in member countries unless it is on the catalogue list. France has shown continued resistance to the introduction of GM seeds, even though the French government has approved their sale. In 2004, six varieties of Monsanto's Bt corn were listed in the French agriculture ministry catalogs, but none were grown until 2006.

In yet another major blow to the biotech industry, French President Nicolas Sarkozy banned a strain of Monsanto GM corn in January 2008. In doing so, he invoked the precautionary principle in light of serious doubts raised about the Monsanto seeds by a scientific panel convened by the French government. France has seen an increase in protest attacks on field crop trials since GM seeds were planted there. In August of 2007, French protestors ripped up crops in a Monsanto corn field, costing the company an estimated 100,000 euros.[9]

Attacks on GM crops are common in other European countries as well. Also in 2007, another biotech company planted a test crop of GM potatoes near Cambridge, England. Despite a security fence, guards, and a court injunction, the plants were destroyed in an overnight raid.[10] The Cambridge crop trial was one of only two expected in Britain that year. The second trial was stopped when environmental activists publicized the location of the field. The company tried to shift to another area, but neighboring farmers protested, fearing the GM seeds and possible contamination of their crops.

This angered American biotech companies, U.S. government officials, and pro-GM farmers, who say that repeated acts of violence and the lack of EU support severely damage American interests and exports. Indeed, trade figures between the United States and the European Union paint a depressing picture for American farmers: "In 1998 U.S. farmers lost about $200 million worth of corn sales to the EU, as exports plummeted to 3 million bushels, down from nearly 70 million in 1997."[11] Corn is the most widely grown crop in the United States, and the United States is also the world's largest grower of corn. Along with cotton and soy, corn is one of the most successful genetically modified crops to date.

International supporters of GM foods argue that the European Union's approach heightens unfounded fears and paints a hypothetical picture of worst-case scenarios. They say this frightens consumers away from GM foods. The battles rage on, and as increasing numbers of large U.S. agricultural exporters adopt GMOs, it is more expensive and difficult for European farmers to avoid them. The harsh reality of dollars and cents may eventually influence the outcome of the GM debate.

The negative reaction to GM foods in Europe may have been caused by the discovery of mad cow disease, or bovine spongiform encephalopathy (BSE), in England. The epidemic in the United Kingdom peaked around 1993, when 1,000 new diseased cows were being reported each week. Over four million cattle were eventually slaughtered to stop the spread of the disease. Scientists theorized that the cows contracted BSE when they ate feed that included contaminated organs and parts of other cattle and sheep. The incubation of BSE in cattle takes at least 30 months, and because most cows are slaughtered by 18 months, meat from infected cows entered the food market undetected. Great Britain and the European Union have now passed strict guidelines preventing the feeding of meat and bone meal to cattle; the United States has not passed the same guidelines. By 2006, there were at least three confirmed cases of BSE in cows in the United States.

In 1996, scientific evidence revealed a link between the consumption of meat from cows with BSE and the incurable brain-wasting disease in humans called variant Creutzfeldt-Jakob disease (vCJD). Since 1995, more than 140 Britons have been diagnosed with vCJD. The number of people ultimately affected by this slow-acting, fatal disease is still being calculated. Researchers have determined that all cases of transmissible spongiform encephalopathy—the family of infectious diseases that includes BSE and CJD—are caused when misshapen proteins called prions attack the brain.

The mad cow disease epidemic badly damaged the confidence of European consumers. Europeans may have considered untested GMOs the next attack on their food supply. Indeed, critics of GMOs question whether the use of growth hormones, insecticides, GM crops, and antibiotics in cattle feed may contribute to the spread of BSE, especially if GM plants experience random protein changes. In 1997, the European Union adopted the "Novel Foods Regulation," which required special labeling of GM foods if any genetically modified content was detected. The regulation failed to define a percentage standard above which a product had to carry a GM label—a lack of specifics that both supporters and critics of GM foods tried to use to their advantage. The following year, France banned two EU-approved GM seed varieties, and other countries followed.

In the fall of 1998, approval of the new biotechnology came to a halt in Europe. Earlier that year, a leading UK researcher, Arpad Pusztai, spoke in a televised interview about the results of a government-commissioned study he conducted on GM potatoes. He stated that the GM potatoes caused damage to the immune systems of rats. Pusztai, a well-respected biochemist with a 35-year career at the Rowett Research Institute in Scotland, was selected in 1992 to head the government's research team. The goal of the study was to devise safety testing methods to evaluate whether GM potatoes had any effect on the nutrition or health of rats. The study was expected to advance to human participants. According to Pusztai, "at the time we started in 1995, there was not a single scientific publication on the potential health effects of any genetically engineered crops."[12]

Although Pusztai did not anticipate problems, once underway, he noticed that the two genetically transformed potato plants they used had very different compositions. In his 1998 interview, he explained that this suggested that harmful changes could appear unexpectedly in GM plants several generations after the seeds were approved for planting, because transferred genes do not always stay at the same DNA location in which they were originally placed. Pusztai also noted changes in the development of the hearts, livers, kidneys, and brains of the rats. He stopped the study. His subsequent interview ignited outrage from British citizens, lawmakers, and consumer activists. Their anger had already been fueled months earlier by England's Prince Charles and his public criticism of GMOs. In the June 8, 1998 *Daily Telegraph,* Charles urged scientists to stop playing God, arguing that genetic engineering "takes mankind into realms that belong to God and God alone. We simply do not know the long-term consequences for human health and the wider environment of releasing plants bred this way."[13]

The Rowett Research Institute issued a statement a few days after Pusztai's interview, rebutting Pusztai's claims and suggesting that he was confused. They declined to release the study results to the media. Pusztai was relieved of his responsibilities for any EU studies, and he retired at the end of that year. But the chilling effect of his words pushed EU members to call for a moratorium on genetic engineering in June 1999. The problem with StarLink corn came to light in the fall of 2000, and it was another four years, until 2004, before the European Commission authorized any GM products.

SUPPORTERS

Profits were a driving force behind the early development of GMOs. In the 1990s, some big U.S. corporations were struggling with the growing costs of creating new pesticides. They also faced a deadline when older pesticides were due to come off patent, releasing those chemical formulas into the public domain. To company officials, biotechnology looked like a fresh area of untapped growth and profits. New seed patents were now the focus of corporations such as Cargill and Archer Daniel Midland, which together hold patents on 80 percent of the world's grain. The other major players, including Syngenta, DuPont, Monsanto, and Aventis, now control two-thirds of the world's agrochemical market.

The strategy was simple: in the 1990s, the major players aggressively bought small seed companies. By 2001, four corporations sold the majority of GM seeds, with corporate giant Monsanto accounting for almost 91 percent of the GM seeds sold that year.[14] Monsanto, Dekalb, and Ciba-Geigy (later renamed Novartis) all worked to get their Bt corn varieties on the market. By 2006, almost 50 percent of the corn planted in the United States was Monsanto's Bt or Roundup Ready seeds.[15]

In fact, the Monsanto Company has developed more genetically engineered seeds and plants than any other corporation. During the 1990s, it also patented and sold GM varieties of rice, cotton, and soybeans. All these plants are engineered to resist the company's top-selling herbicide, Roundup, now the most profitable herbicide in the world. In 2002, the picture for Monsanto was not so positive; the company had suffered a 65 percent drop in sales of Roundup. But by 2008, thanks to the purchase of seed companies, advances in GMO technology, and the pairing of the seeds with its herbicide, the company posted huge earnings. In January 2008, Monsanto reported annual earnings of over $256 million in the fiscal first quarter, compared to $90 million for the same period in 2007.[16] With the development of corn ethanol on the horizon, the value of Monsanto's stock should continue to climb.

Along with large biotech corporations, other organizations that strongly support GM technology include Sense About Science, the National Center for Food and Agriculture Policy (NCFAP), and Truth about Trade & Technology. Sense About Science is a UK lobby group that was launched in 2002. The Web site refers to a network of scientists who support an evidence-based approach to technological developments. The NCFAP is a private, nonprofit research organization formed in 1992. Consumer advocates have called the organization a pro-GM industry group whose funding for NCFAP biotechnology studies is linked to such donors as Monsanto, Grocery Manufacturers of America, DuPont, Aventis, and the Rockefeller Foundation. Truth about Trade & Technology is based in Iowa, and describes itself on its Web site as a grassroots farm organization and supporter of free trade and agricultural biotechnology. The organization posts a running total of biotech crops planted and harvested around the world on its home page.

OPPONENTS

Opponents of genetically modified foods agree on several basic concepts, most importantly that the benefits of GMOs do not outweigh the risks. At the same time, they worry that the debate over genetically engineered food may distract people from looking at more useful alternatives for solving world hunger. These activists suggest that the world has enough food available, but that it is not distributed fairly. They wonder how the world's poor will find enough resources to buy genetically engineered seeds when they lack money to buy seeds now. Corporations such as Monsanto have shown no willingness to give away free seeds, and they have taken legal action against inadvertent cross-pollination.

Opponents of genetic engineering argue that it will not address the problems of income disparity, and that ending poverty and political inequality is the only way to stop world hunger.

The largest groups opposed to genetically engineered foods include Greenpeace, the Center for Food Safety (CFS), the Alliance for Bio-Integrity, GM Watch, and the Union of Concerned Scientists. Greenpeace has offices in 40 countries across Europe, the Americas, Asia, and the Pacific. The group started in 1971 when a team of individuals took a small fishing boat to sea to protect endangered animals off the coast of Alaska. Since that time, they have grown into an international advocate for the environment, working to change attitudes and behavior, to protect and conserve the environment, and to promote peace.

Greenpeace officially applauds scientific progress on molecular biology when it believes such progress is used to increase understanding of nature and provide new medical tools. But Greenpeace members criticize the untested use of genetically modified organisms as a giant genetic experiment by commercial interests. They advocate immediate labeling of GM ingredients, and the segregation of GM crops from conventional seeds. Greenpeace also continues to demand advanced scientific testing of GMOs, of their impact on the environment, and of their potential to damage human health.

The Alliance for Bio-Integrity was founded by lawyer Stephen M. Drucker, who played a key role in the 1998 lawsuit against the FDA. The CFS is a nonprofit, public interest environmental advocacy organization that began in 1997 for the direct purpose of challenging GM food technologies and promoting alternatives. The organization has offices in Washington DC and San Francisco. The CFS joined the 1998 lawsuit against the FDA along with the Alliance for Bio-Integrity. In June 2006, the CFS filed another suit against the FDA to force the government to require labels and identify any foods with GM components. GM Watch was founded in 1998 in Norfolk, UK, in response to growing international concern about genetic engineering, and now has contacts in several European countries. A private, nonprofit organization, GM Watch specifically functions to publicly question the genetic engineering industry.

THE FUTURE

Webster's Dictionary defines controversies as discussions of questions in which opposing opinions clash. Few would deny that the controversy over genetically engineered foods is a clash of both political and scientific opinions. On one side are those who demand the right to know what they are eating. They call genetically modified foods an experiment in progress with unknown consequences. On the other side are corporations, governments, and scientists, who say no evidence of harm has come to light, and argue that the use of biotechnology is imperative to feed a hungry world. Although GMO research that will improve health and nutrition has not kept pace with the research and development of plants that resist pests or tolerate herbicides, there are new products said to be in the advanced stages of development. These include oils with fewer fatty acids, grains with increased protein content, and various plants with higher vitamin and mineral levels.

Consumers must ask themselves whether this technology is being pushed to the market before risks are understood and managed. Opponents use the examples of DDT and polychlorinated biphenyls (PCBs), both sold before they were adequately tested. The human health costs and environmental damage these substances created by the time they were banned was huge. For consumers wary of GM products, the best choice is to eat foods with the certified organic label. Thanks to the Organic Foods Production Act of 1990 (OFPA), there is a uniform organic standard in place for farmers.

The OFPA is enforced by the USDA, and although the agency proposed rules over the years to permit irradiated foods and biotech foods, the organic standard ultimately adopted in 2002 explicitly excludes any GM foods. Although it was not designed to assist consumers looking to avoid genetically modified foods, for now the label's net effect means no GM ingredients are used in organic products.

Another strategy for consumers wishing to avoid GM products is to scan labels for common GM ingredients such as corn oil, corn syrup, cornstarch, soy protein, soy oil, soy sauce, lecithin, cottonseed oil, and canola oil. An FDA report published in 2000 listed those foods among many that tested positive for the presence of unlabeled genetically modified ingredients. The FDA list also included various well known items: Duncan Hines cake mix, Jiffy corn muffin mix, Ultra Slim Fast, Aunt Jemima Pancake Mix, and Kellogg's Corn Flakes to name a few. For shoppers who want information on GM-free foods, the "True Food Shopping List" from the Greenpeace Web site provides a list of foods without GM ingredients.

Humankind is capable of using invention to control and direct the future, but to achieve a better and safer world it must be done carefully. It may all come down to education and the free flow of information for consumers, who will ultimately decide to accept or reject genetically modified foods.

CHAPTER 6

Vitamins and Supplements: A Love-Hate Relationship

Americans are bombarded with conflicting reports about the benefits of this and the harmful effects of that. We bounce from diet to diet, and indulge in junk food and fast food to the exclusion of almost anything else. Our foods are packed with fats, calories, salt, high-fructose corn syrup, and chemicals, but little that's good for us. Enter the "magic bullets" of vitamins and supplements. Yet before Americans pop a pill or take a tablet, they may want to educate themselves on the health and safety issues that vitamins and supplements present, and on the research that is just beginning to illuminate their long-term effects.

Multivitamins and supplements have been around for over 50 years, and are considered by many Americans to be a form of nutritional insurance, a way to make up for bad eating habits. Today, they comprise a multibillion-dollar industry. According to *Nutrition Business Journal,* a market research publication that tracks the supplement industry, the total sales figure for vitamins and supplements in the United States in 2006 was a whopping $22 billion.[1]

The American Dietetic Association (ADA) suggests that vitamins and supplements may be necessary for some people based on their specific circumstances, including pregnant women; nursing mothers; vegans; people with food allergies or food disease, such as celiac disease; people with cancer or bone disease; and senior citizens. What about adults and children who do not fit into these categories? Does everyone really need vitamins and supplements?

Surprisingly, the 2005 *Dietary Guidelines for Americans* does not recommend any vitamin supplement for a healthy population consuming a variety of foods. The guidelines are updated every five years. The ADA echoed that finding, saying "there is little scientific evidence of benefit to the average person" from a low-dose multivitamin or multivitamin and mineral supplement.[2]

By contrast, the Council for Responsible Nutrition (CRN), the Vitamin C Foundation, The National Health Federation (NHF), and the International Society for Orthomolecular Medicine (ISOM) are among the many organizations strongly promoting the use of vitamins and other key supplements and offering their own evidence of the health benefits.

TOP TEN SUPPLEMENTS

Americans may be overwhelmed by conflicting information, but they continue to swallow dietary supplements in increasing numbers, according to survey results released by the Council for Responsible Nutrition (CRN) in October 2007. The CRN is the supplement industry's leading trade association. Their online survey, undertaken by market researcher Ipsos-Public Affairs, found that 52 percent of Americans say they are regular users of dietary supplements. That number is up from 46 percent in 2006.[3]

The top ten popular supplement categories people are using, based on yearly sales figures and compiled by *Nutrition Business Journal,* include multivitamins, meal replacements, sports nutrition supplements, calcium, B vitamins, vitamin C, glucosamine and chondroitin, homeopathic medicine, vitamin D, and fish oil. Here is a brief introduction to America's most-wanted supplements:

1. *Multivitamins* were first introduced to consumers in the 1950s to offset the effects of an explosion of overprocessed foods. Americans from all walks of life had become more interested in low cost and convenience than in nutrition. In the process, they had filled their kitchens with items like Wonder Bread, a white, fluffy loaf that promised to "build strong bodies 12 ways." The enrichment was necessary because all the bread's original nutrients were processed out of it.

    Multivitamins have come a long way since those early days. Now they are manufactured based on age and sex, from chewable vitamins for children to those designed for seniors, women, and even senior women. They come in all shapes, sizes, and flavors. Although there is little hard scientific data from major medical groups or government agencies to show any substantial benefit from multivitamin use by otherwise healthy children and adults, there are just as many supporters of their benefits in the alternative medicine and dietary supplements communities.

2. *Meal replacements* are marketed to dieters who want to lose weight by substituting diet shakes, bars, or prepackaged meals for their regular foods. However, one important drawback to meal replacements is that they are processed foods; although they contain added vitamins and minerals, they lack fiber, antioxidants, and the other health benefits associated with eating fresh foods, especially fruits and vegetables.
3. *Sports nutrition supplements* include a vast array of powders, drinks, gels, bars, and pills, and contain vitamins, amino acids, minerals, herbs, and other botanicals. These products were developed for serious athletes, but are routinely purchased and used by everyone from recreational athletes to couch potatoes. Sport drinks are especially popular. Unfortunately, studies have shown that they are more acidic than orange juice and may contribute to the erosion of tooth enamel. They often contain high amounts of sodium and caffeine, which is a factor in lower calcium levels, because calcium is excreted through urine and both salt and caffeine greatly increase urine output.

    In fact, our national intake of caffeine and sodium is sky-high. The latest report from the Institute of Medicine suggests that the average American eats about 4,000 milligrams (mg) of sodium a day. The Institute recommends only 1,500 mg of sodium a day, and 1,200 mg for anyone over 70. Americans also consume about 45 million pounds of caffeine each year in the form of coffee, soft drinks, food, and drugs.
4. *Calcium* is the next most popular dietary supplement in this country, and is most often lacking in the average American diet. Given the high number of Americans who eat and drink excessive amounts of sodium and caffeine, Americans likely lack calcium in part due to the diuretic effects of our daily food and beverage choices.
5. The *B vitamins* include B1 or thiamine, B2 or riboflavin, B3 or niacin, B5 or pantothenic acid, B6 or pyridoxine, B7 or biotin, B9 or folic acid, and B12. Most people do not need vitamin B supplements, and overuse can create problems. Vitamin B3, also known as niacin, is used to lower cholesterol, but it can also cause liver damage and prevent the absorption of medications if too much is taken. It should only be used under a doctor's supervision. Vitamin B6 has been promoted in the treatment of everything from depression to premenstrual syndrome (PMS). However, even doses less than 500 milligrams per day may cause nerve damage and numbness in the arms and legs.

Vitamin B9, also known as folic acid, has been added to all enriched food products, such as breads, cereals, flours, pasta, and other grains, since 1996. That was the year the Food and Drug Administration (FDA) required bakers to add enough folic acid to enriched white flour to raise the average intake by an estimated 70 to 120 micrograms a day. Since 1996, instances of neural tube birth defects such as spina bifida and anencephaly have dropped in this country. However, researchers now worry that an overabundance of folic acid may raise the risk of colon cancer or accelerate other forms of cancer like leukemia. Vitamin B12 deficiencies are rare, but adults over age 50 do have a reduced ability to absorb it. Unfortunately, folic acid can make a B12 deficiency worse, and can cause anemia. Doctors recommend not taking folic acid and B12 together to prevent this situation.

6. Americans can thank Dr. Linus Pauling, a two-time Nobel Prize winner, for our love affair with *vitamin C*. At age 65, when most people consider retirement, Pauling began his research on the therapeutic effects of vitamin C. He published his opinions in 1970 in a book titled *Vitamin C and the Common Cold.* In the book, he claimed that large amounts of vitamin C will cure the common cold and some forms of cancer. There is still no definitive scientific proof that megadoses of vitamin C have any benefits, and many scientists argue that excess intake of the vitamin is a waste of money and may actually be harmful. Still, when a cold strikes, many consumers take vitamin C.

7. The combination of *glucosamine and chondroitin* is sold as a one-two punch for people suffering from arthritis and joint pain. But these supplements, taken alone or in combination, were not found to provide significant relief from osteoarthritis pain in a study published in the *New England Journal of Medicine*.[4] Word of mouth keeps these supplements on the bestsellers list.

8. *Homeopathy*, or homeopathic medicine, is a medical philosophy dating back to the late 1700s, and was founded by Dr. Samuel Christian Friedrich Hahnemann. Based on the idea that our bodies have a self-healing response to illness and injury, the theory suggests that if a substance causes symptoms when given to a healthy person, a small dose may cure a sick person with the same symptoms. The Web site of the National Institute of Health's (NIH) National Center for Complementary and Alternative Medicine notes that studies on the success of homeopathy are contradictory.

9. *Vitamin D* is an essential vitamin manufactured in the skin during exposure to the sun. It is fat-soluble, and responsible for regulating

the absorption and use of calcium and phosphorous in a healthy person. This vitamin also helps build normal bones, cartilage, and teeth. It can be manufactured in the body with as little as a half-hour of sunlight. Unfortunately, vitamin D is highly toxic, and excessive consumption can cause nausea, loss of appetite, and kidney damage. Prolonged use of megadoses may result in kidney failure and death.
10. *Omega-3 fatty acids* are a booming supplement, sold for the prevention of heart disease. The American Heart Association (AHA) recommends eating fatty fish twice weekly as part of a heart-healthy diet, prompting many consumers to turn to daily fish oil supplements. However, there is no definitive scientific evidence that omega-3 oil supplements have any benefit in healthy individuals. Unfortunately, researchers are concerned that excessive fish oil consumption, whether from natural sources or supplements, may increase the risk of stroke and weaken the immune system.

LEGISLATION

At this point average American consumers, confused by conflicting information, may turn to the government for reassurance that supplements and vitamins are safe, effective, and truthfully advertised. They will be disappointed. Although some aspects of marketing are regulated, federal oversight and the ability to regulate dietary supplements was severely curtailed in 1994, when Congress passed the Dietary Supplement Health and Education Act (DSHEA).

The new law, which amended the Federal Food, Drug, and Cosmetic Act, created a regulatory framework for the safety and labeling of dietary supplements, defined them as a separate category of products, and dramatically changed how they would be handled. Unlike the earlier laws that protected American consumers from fraudulent products, this law turned the burden of proof back on the FDA. Now dietary supplement manufacturers do not have to prove that their product is safe before it can be sold. Instead, the government must wait for reports of dangerous complications. The FDA must also provide overwhelming evidence from clinical trials and reports of harm before they can force a product off the shelves. Manufacturers of prescription drugs, by law, must still prove their products are safe before they are sold to the public.

The DSHEA further defines dietary supplements as products that are intended to supplement the diet; contain one or more ingredients such as vitamins, herbs, or amino acids; are intended to be taken by mouth; are labeled as dietary supplements; are produced in a quality manner; do not contain contaminants or impurities; and are accurately labeled. Although the DSHEA does not allow supplement labels to claim that supplements prevent, cure, or treat disease, labels are allowed to carry claims that the product supports some body structure or function. For example, supplement labels cannot say a product prevents heart disease, but they can say it promotes heart health. They cannot say the product prevents colds, but they can say it supports a healthy immune system. Although supplement makers are supposed to formulate their products according to defined chemical criteria and make sure the products contain just what the labels describe, neither the government nor the industry sets any meaningful standards for their actual contents.

A prime example of how DSHEA has weakened the government's ability to protect consumers against harmful supplements is the story of ephedra. Products with ephedra were finally banned in the United States after almost 10 years of being linked to growing numbers of heart attacks, strokes, seizures, and deaths. The ephedra plant, known as Ma Huang in Chinese, had been used for centuries by the ancient Chinese to treat coughs, colds, fever, sweating, congestion, shortness of breath, and water retention. The herb was processed into a drug called ephedrine that appeared in the United States in weight-loss formulas. The FDA banned the combination of ephedrine and caffeine in 1983 based on growing concerns about the safety of that drug mixture. Problems continued because even though the two ingredients together were illegal, ephedra, the natural herb, was still legal in the United States.

Because ephedra was classified as an herb and not a drug, its use in diet pills continued, along with its potentially deadly consequences. Finally, in 2003, it appeared that ephedra might have played a role in the death of Baltimore Orioles pitcher Steve Bechler. The ensuing public outrage helped the FDA push through a ban on ephedra in March 2004. But ephedra is not gone yet; an appeal was filed in 2006 challenging the ban, and may still work its way to the U.S. Supreme Court. Ephedra makers continue to insist that the herb is safe when used as directed.

Congress did respond to concerns about how difficult it was for the FDA to ban ephedra sales even after thousands of people suffered serious health problems. They passed the Dietary Supplement and Nonprescription Drug Consumer Protection Act in December 2006. The act mandates that manufacturers of dietary supplements and nonprescription drugs must notify the FDA about serious adverse problems related to their products, especially deaths, life-threatening events, hospitalizations, significant disabilities, birth defects, or the need for medical intervention based on their products. Manufacturers are also required to add a contact telephone number or address to their product labels for consumers.

NATURAL PROBLEMS

Too many people find it hard to believe that something labeled "natural" can be harmful. Unfortunately, the more than 10,000 people who became ill and the 38 who died from the amino acid L-tryptophan in 1989 are proof that natural, in some cases, is also deadly. Tryptophan is an amino acid that normally helps control the brain chemical serotonin, and affects sleep, mood, and appetite. It is most easily recognized as the ingredient in milk or turkey responsible for a sleepy feeling after a turkey dinner or a glass of warm milk at bedtime. Isolated as a nutritional supplement, it was incorporated into pills and sold in health food stores under a variety of brand names.

Once sales of the supplement began in the late 1980s, people across the country developed debilitating symptoms, including muscle weakness, pain spasms, high fevers, and rashes. The common link was L-tryptophan. The problem was eventually traced back to a batch of L-tryptophan from one of the largest chemical companies in Japan. The pills were manufactured after the company had substantially changed its production process. The company had also used genetically engineered bacteria in the production of the drug. Opponents of genetic engineering suggested that the engineered bacteria may have caused the problem. Another theory focused on a recently installed filtration system, which may have let through toxic impurities; the same toxic compounds were discovered in batches of unmodified bacteria used by other manufacturers of L-tryptophan. As more and more people got sick and the common link was clearly established, doctors theorized that some people were more susceptible to L-tryptophan eosinophilia myalgia syndrome (EMS), as a reaction to the pure amino acid. Sadly, the Japanese batch made a reaction more likely. The company destroyed the modified bacteria.

Although L-tryptophan is now banned in the United States, other amino acids remain on the shelves. There are also new supplements for sale that label themselves alternatives to L-tryptophan; they are marketed as antidepressants, as sleep aids, and for weight loss. New cases of EMS were reported in 2002, and the FDA suggested that anyone taking these newer products remain vigilant and watch for EMS symptoms.

What if L-tryptophan had been named a drug instead of a supplement? First, its manufacturers would have been required to perform detailed studies of possible risks. Second, the manufacturing process would have been closely regulated, and the plants would have been inspected. As a supplement, L-tryptophan faced none of those safeguards.

However, the FDA did try to take amino acids off the shelves before the L-trytophan crisis. As early as 1976, the FDA attempted to set limits on the potency of vitamins and certain supplements. Their efforts triggered an avalanche of letters and calls protesting any changes. The reaction from the supplement industry and angry consumers was so strong that it resulted in passage of the Proxmire Amendment. Named after the bill's chief sponsor, Senator William Proxmire of Wisconsin, the legislation prohibited the FDA from putting limits on the potency of vitamins and minerals in food supplements, or, more importantly, from regulating them as drugs based on their potency. Congress made sure vitamins and supplements would not be regulated without clear and substantial proof of real danger.

More Bad News

Unfortunately, L-trytophan is not the only example of death and devastation from a supplement; kidney failure and bladder cancer were the side effects of the herb aristolochia. In 1994, a growing number of patients from a Belgian weight loss clinic developed severe kidney disease. By the time the herb aristolochia was identified as the culprit, there were 105 documented cases of rapid kidney failure. Some 30 of the women died, and at least half of the rest had to have kidney transplants. The herb and its derivative, aristolochic acid, were quickly banned in seven European countries, as well as in Egypt, Japan, Canada, and Venezuela. The FDA acted within the scope of its powers, and in May 2000 wrote a letter to manufacturers and distributors, "urging" them to stop selling supplements containing aristolochic acid. By the time the FDA wrote a second letter, again asking companies to stop selling the dangerous herb, at least two new cases of kidney failure linked to aristolochia were reported in the United States. That number may be larger, but public health departments across the country suggest there is no way to pinpoint the actual number of cases of aristolochic acid poisoning in this country.

How can it be that this ancient Chinese herb was never found to be toxic before? Apparently one of its most insidious features is that damage or illness occurs years after the herb is taken. The delayed symptoms kept people from understanding its toxicity until the Belgian doctors linked the pieces together. An editorial published in the June 2004 issue of the journal *Nephrology* described the hundreds of cases that were now being linked to aristolochic acid poisoning in China. The director of the renal division of Peking University First Hospital in Beijing added more bad news: aristolochic acid is extremely carcinogenic, so patients who survived the initial crisis could face cancer.

Aristolochic acid is still available through the internet according to an article in the *New England Journal of Medicine*. The article reported about 100 Web sites selling 115 products believed to contain the herb, many labeled "natural" and ranging from cough syrups to products for PMS.[5] A 2006 study in *Clinical Toxicology* examined raw herbs purchased from Chinese wholesalers, and found that four of the six contained aristolochic acid; of seven manufactured products examined, two contained it as well. This raised serious concerns about the safety of Chinese herbal remedies. Researchers suggested lax regulatory controls, widespread misidentification, and incorrect herbs substituted by suppliers as key reasons for the problem.[6]

Consumers should not expect action from the FDA any time soon to fix this dangerous situation. In a series of reports detailed in the *New York Times* on January 29, 2008, the Government Accountability Office (GAO) described the FDA as overwhelmed by a flood of imports. The report included a recent assessment by the GAO's Science Board, which concluded that the FDA is so broken down that it is "incapable of protecting the public."[7]

TRUE BELIEVERS

Of course, there are Americans who believe that these tales of doom and gloom are exaggerations—or worse, part of a government plan to rob citizens of easy access to vitamins and supplements. Chief among those critics is the International Society for Orthomolecular Medicine (ISOM). Dr. Linus Pauling, chemist and Nobel laureate, is regarded by some as the founder of the science of orthomolecular medicine. He introduced the word "orthomolecular" in the 1960s to describe the use of natural substances, especially nutrients, in treating illness and maintaining good health.

Pauling and several colleagues founded the Institute of Orthomolecular Medicine, later renamed the Linus Pauling Institute of Science and Medicine, in Palo Alto, California. According to the ISOM Web site, orthomolecular treatments include "dietary manipulation, nutrition supplementation, herbal remedies, homeopathic treatments, detoxification and safe forms of megavitamin therapy." The megadoses used in "megavitamin" therapy are defined in scientific terms as doses that are 10 times the Recommended Dietary Allowance (RDA) or more.

The ISOM Web site contains case studies that the group claims demonstrate the effectiveness of their practices. Andrew W. Saul, PhD, editor-in-chief of the Orthomolecular Medicine News Service, has routinely criticized the media for accepting and promoting all government-sponsored studies showing harmful effects from supplements. He wrote on his personal web site, "The sky is not falling. Vitamins save lives. We are a nation of sick, under-nourished, and over-medicated people. Vitamins are not the problem; they are the solution."[8]

The Council for Responsible Nutrition (CRN) likewise claims that vitamins and supplements help prevent disease. This trade association was founded in 1973 and now includes some 70 member companies, among them Archer Daniels Midland Company, Bayer Corporation, Shaklee Corporation, and Cargill Health and Food Technologies. The CRN continuously lobbies against any new FDA regulatory controls over vitamins or other supplements. On their Web site, they rank their ability to maintain and improve consumer confidence in their members' products as a top priority. Recent links focused on the positive effects of vitamin D in lowering cancer risks for older women, and on the potential helpful effects of increased vitamin D on lowering blood pressure. This increase in vitamin D according to the CRN may decrease blood pressure for people who suffer from hypertension.

While Pauling focused on establishing orthomolecular medicine, other medical doctors developed their own work with supplements. Dr. Robert C. Atkins, famous for his protein-rich diet, advocated taking 20 nutritional supplements a day; he personally took 60 daily. Atkins first appeared on the national stage in 1973 with the publication of his high-protein, low-carbohydrate eating plan. His book, *Dr. Atkins' Diet Revolution* (1972), quickly became a bestseller.

After the success of his book, Atkins opened an alternative healing clinic and continued to publish books. His first book dealing with alternative healing, *Dr. Atkins' Nutrition Breakthrough: How to Treat Your Medical Condition without Drugs,* was published in 1981. In 1998, he released *Dr. Atkins' Vita-Nutrient Solution: Nature's Answer to Drugs.* Atkins's work with supplements was honored by the National Health Federation (NHF), and he received their Man of the Year Award. Established in 1955, the NHF is an international consumer education and health freedom organization. According to its Web site, members "work to protect individuals' rights to choose to consume healthy food, take supplements, and use alternative therapies without government restrictions."[9]

It was biochemist Irwin Stone who introduced Linus Pauling to the value of vitamin C in preventing colds. Stone suggested that by treating vitamin C, or ascorbic acid, as a nutrient with a minimum daily requirement instead of a crucial enzyme, people were living in a state of disease he named hypoascorbemia. He believed that people receive only one or two percent of the amount of ascorbic acid they need to be healthy. Stone published his research and findings in 1972, in a book titled *The Healing Factor: Vitamin C against Disease.*

Pauling credited Stone's research for his own developing ideas, and wrote the foreword for Stone's book along with Dr. Albert Szent-Gyorgyi, recipient of the 1937 Nobel Prize for his discovery of vitamin C. Szent-Gyorgyi, who originally gave vitamin C the name ascorbic acid, is also credited as being the first to suggest its use in treating cancer. Szent-Gyorgyi was 80 years old when he founded the National Foundation for Cancer Research in 1973. The NFCR is still active and supports cancer research, as well as public education on the prevention, early diagnosis, treatment, and continuing search for a cure for cancer.

New Studies

The potential curative effect of vitamins on cancer has been debated for decades by scientists and doctors, including Pauling, Szent-Gyorgyi, and Stone. Researchers are now working with new studies that examine whether vitamins *promote* cancer growth if taken in large doses. Joel Mason, director of the Vitamins and Carcinogenesis Laboratory at the Jean Mayer USDA Human Nutrition Research Center on Aging at Tufts University, recently published data showing that colorectal cancer rates rose soon after companies started adding folic acid to foods in the 1990s.[10]

There are theories to explain this early data showing over 15,000 extra cases of colorectal cancer per year. Mason suggested that small doses of folic acid may protect against colorectal cancer, but he cautioned, "we started seeing that an abundant quantity of folic acid might accelerate carcinogenesis in animal studies, and now data from human studies is starting to emerge."[11] Folic acid is necessary for the synthesis of DNA, and cells produce DNA every time they divide. For people who have cancer or precancerous cells, excessive folic acid may increase the body's ability to produce DNA and feed the cancer cells. Whereas foods rich in folate are not a problem because the human body absorbs the folate less efficiently, supplements and fortified foods can quickly bring folate levels to over 800 micrograms of folic acid—double the RDA of 400 micrograms per day.

Another nutrient getting a hard look under the microscope is selenium. A study developed to test whether selenium lowers the risk of squamous and basal cell skin cancers found no protective value. In 2003, studies showed a slight increase in squamous cell skin cancers with selenium, according to James Marshall of the Roswell Park Cancer Institute in Buffalo, New York, who headed up the study. In another unexpected result, Marshall noted that after nearly eight years of the study, there were more diagnoses of diabetes among selenium takers than among those taking the placebo.[12] Adding to the concern, a study of some 9,000 U.S. residents published in *Diabetes Care* in 2007 found that diabetes was more common in people with higher blood selenium levels. Marshall cautioned consumers against taking selenium supplements without checking with their physician. The Daily Value for selenium recommended by the FDA is 70 micrograms. Daily Values are reference numbers developed by the FDA to help consumers determine healthy amounts of various nutrients.

BUYERS BEWARE?

The science of dietary supplements is ambiguous. Clinical trials compare one group taking a supplement or vitamin to another group taking placebos, and track those groups to see what conclusions they can draw. Supplement industry officials like to interpret the results in their favor, whereas the government acts to protect consumers. Everyone sees something different in the results. If you are like the majority of Americans, you may take a vitamin or supplement of one kind or another. Will vitamins or supplements help those who skip meals, eat out too often, or don't get the recommended amounts of fruits, vegetables, and fiber? Americans think they will, and they assume that vitamins and supplements are safe. Consumers, along with their physicians, should decide whether they need supplements and which ones to take. Services like MedWatch—the FDA Safety Information and Adverse Event Reporting Program—will help keep Americans aware of safety alerts, recalls, withdrawals, and important labeling changes. Whatever the decision, the best advice is still found in the Latin phrase *caveat emptor*—"let the buyer beware."

CHAPTER 7

Vegetarians: You Are What You Eat

Hot dogs, hamburgers, bacon, and beef: it doesn't get more American when it comes to food. Add in chicken nuggets, sausage, ham, and all other meats, and figures from the U.S. Department of Agriculture (USDA) show that per capita meat consumption for the average American in 2007 was 273 pounds.[1] We are the world's leaders in eating meat, a distinction that raises some important health questions. For example, red meat is one of the first foods doctors advise patients to stop eating if they are at risk of heart disease, because of its high levels of cholesterol. Red meat has also been linked to an increased risk of arthritis and bowel cancer in recent studies.

While no one is suggesting that eating meat automatically causes cancer, it is interesting to note that Americans have the world's highest risk of developing cancer. Statistics show that U.S. citizens have about an 18 percent probability of developing cancer before age 65—almost double that of other countries such as Japan, where citizens have a 10 percent chance according to data from the Centers for Disease Control and Prevention (CDC).[2]

What's a meat lover to do? One option, according to the American Dietetic Association (ADA), the American Heart Association, the National Cancer Institute, and the U.S. Department of Health and Human Services, is to strike a better balance in the American diet: five fruits and vegetables a day, along with protein from a variety of sources instead of just from meat. In fact, all these organizations now support a well-planned vegetarian diet, and want Americans to strongly consider eating some meatless meals. In a 2003 position paper, the ADA called appropriately planned vegetarian diets "healthful and nutritionally adequate," and said they "provide health benefits in the prevention and treatment of certain diseases."[3]

Americans may actually be listening to that advice. The ranks of celebrity vegetarians now include Chelsea Clinton, Gwyneth Paltrow, and Brad Pitt, along with musicians Prince, Michael Jackson, Alanis Morissette, and Justin Timberlake. At the same time, the number of average Americans who eliminate animal products from their diets is visibly growing. The Vegetarian Resource Group (VRG), a nonprofit educational organization, conducted a national poll in 2006 to determine how many Americans follow a vegetarian diet. They discovered that 2.8 percent of adults aged 18 years or older say they never eat meat, fish, or fowl and consider themselves vegetarian. An even higher proportion, 6.7 percent, never eat red meat. This is an increase from the 2000 poll. Using those 2000 U.S. census figures, the VRG estimates that there are more than five million adult vegetarians in the United States.[4]

VEGETARIAN BY MANY NAMES

Vegetarian is a blanket term for a person whose diet omits animal products. However, there are many definitions and categories, from the very stringent to the most lenient. It's important to remember that vegetarianism is a personal choice and is best defined by each individual and his or her specific dietary needs. In the most basic sense, a vegetarian is a person who does not eat meat, poultry, fish, or any kind of animal product. Vegetarians do eat fruits, vegetables, legumes, grains, soy, seeds, and nuts.

Subclassifications include vegans, lacto-vegetarians, ovo-vegetarians, pollo-vegetarians, pesca-vegetarians, and lacto-ovo-vegetarians. The lacto-vegetarian has a diet that includes dairy foods but not eggs. The reverse is the ovo-vegetarian, who eats eggs but no dairy. Both lacto- and ovo-vegetarians do not eat meat, poultry, or fish products. The lacto-ovo-vegetarian consumes milk, cheese, yogurt, and eggs but not meat, fish, or poultry. This designation is the easiest eating style in terms of menu planning, and usually offers the largest variety of choices for those dining in sit-down or fast-food restaurants. Most vegetarians in the United States are lacto-ovo-vegetarians, according to the ADA.

A pollo-vegetarian eats a diet similar to that of a lacto-ovo-vegetarian, but also includes poultry among food selections. The pesca-vegetarian mimics the lacto-ovo eating habits but includes fish and seafood. The strictest category is the vegan, who avoids all animal products, including hidden items such as gelatin, beef and chicken stocks, lard, and, for many vegans, honey. A vegan diet includes vegetables, fruits, grains, legumes, nuts, and seeds. Many vegans also avoid products such as wool, leather, silk, and cosmetics and soaps made from animals.

HISTORY OF VEGETARIANISM

Today's vegetarians find themselves in good company no matter what eating style they prefer. The vegetarian community through history has included the likes of Albert Einstein, Benjamin Franklin, Charles Darwin, Leonardo da Vinci, Vincent van Gogh, Abraham Lincoln, Mahatma Gandhi, Thomas Edison, and Henry David Thoreau. British vegetarian Colin Spencer, in his book *The Heretic's Feast: A History of Vegetarianism,* traced meatless eating back to Greek philosopher Pythagoras, who told followers that a diet without meat was natural and sensible. In fact, until the nineteenth century, vegetarians were known as Pythagoreans. Pythagoras is famous for developing the Pythagorean theorem in mathematics and for his discovery of irrational numbers, and was the first Greek philosopher to suggest the existence of the soul. To support his beliefs, he founded a philosophical and religious school. The students at Pythagoras's school were required to eat a vegetarian diet due to his belief that all souls come from the same source and all living things are related through a kinship of nature.

Pythagoras was an original thinker who brought together knowledge of the different cultures he studied, from Egypt to Babylon and further East. Vegetarianism has been practiced for centuries in the East, where practitioners of the Hindu religion make up the largest concentration of vegetarians in the world. The tradition of vegetarianism in India includes the belief that cows are sacred creatures with souls. It also connects to the idea of karma—the notion that previous acts determine what animal the soul will inhabit during the process of rebirth, a process that has no beginning or end but is instead part of a perpetual cycle to become one with God. Buddhism, like Hinduism, also rejects eating meat, and teaches compassion toward all creatures and all forms of life based on the belief that rebirth is infinite and can lead to a higher rebirth as a human or god.

The vegetarian ethic slowly spread during the seventeenth century, according to Spencer. The New World was discovered, and with it a native culture that prayed for the spirit of an animal before it was hunted and killed. Native Americans believed in a world shared by all creatures and nurtured by Mother Earth. Later, in Europe, Thomas Tryon—one of England's most outspoken vegetarians—publicly supported a meatless diet. Tryon was born in 1634, and by age 11 was tending sheep for his father. As an adult, Tryon's influence extended across the Atlantic Ocean to

Americans such as Benjamin Franklin. Tryon's book, *The Way to Health, Long Life and Happiness, Or a Discourse of Temperance,* apparently converted Franklin to vegetarianism at the age of sixteen. Franklin wrote in his autobiography that he saved money and found more time to study by not eating meat. As an adult, Franklin eventually returned meat to his diet.

For the upper classes, the eighteenth century was a time of meat-eating gluttony, overweight, and the diseases of obesity. However, by the end of the century, one of America's early notable vegetarians emerged. Sylvester Graham advocated a high-fiber, natural-food diet to cure cholera, alcoholism, and a host of digestive ills. He was born in 1794 in Connecticut, and like many other health reformers had an early history of bad health. Graham was the youngest of 17 children, and his father, Massachusetts minister John Graham, died when he was just two years old. His mother was unable to care for the children, and he was passed from relative to relative for years.

Graham, ordained as a minister in 1826, most famously offered the advice that thick, coarse bread baked at home and eaten daily must be the mainstay of a healthy diet. This thick bread was the early version of today's graham cracker. Graham decided that eating this whole wheat bread instead of white bread and avoiding too much salt, meat, and fat would effectively treat constipation, stomachaches, and other chronic illnesses that plagued many Americans. He was named president of the American Vegetarian Society, founded in 1849 in New York City. The society's membership included Harriet Beecher Stowe and journalist Horace Greeley.

Graham recognized that diet and health were directly connected long before the discovery of nutrition, fiber, vitamins, minerals, and cholesterol. He died in 1851, but his influence on the American diet and on vegetarianism continued. Per capita meat consumption began to decline as Americans ate more fresh fruit and vegetables and better-balanced meals. Graham moved public opinion away from gluttony and poor digestion toward eating for good health.

Meat consumption remained low for much of the twentieth century, because working-class people could not afford beef, chicken, or pork on a regular basis. It wasn't until the business of animal agriculture brought down the price of meat that average Americans added it to their daily diet. By the 1960s, Americans had substantially increased their daily consumption of meat, but at the same time they moved away from the local butcher. Now shoppers flocked to neighborhood supermarkets to pick up packages that bore no resemblance to the original animal. The neighborhood butcher was soon obsolete, even as the demand for meat continued to grow and the prices dropped.

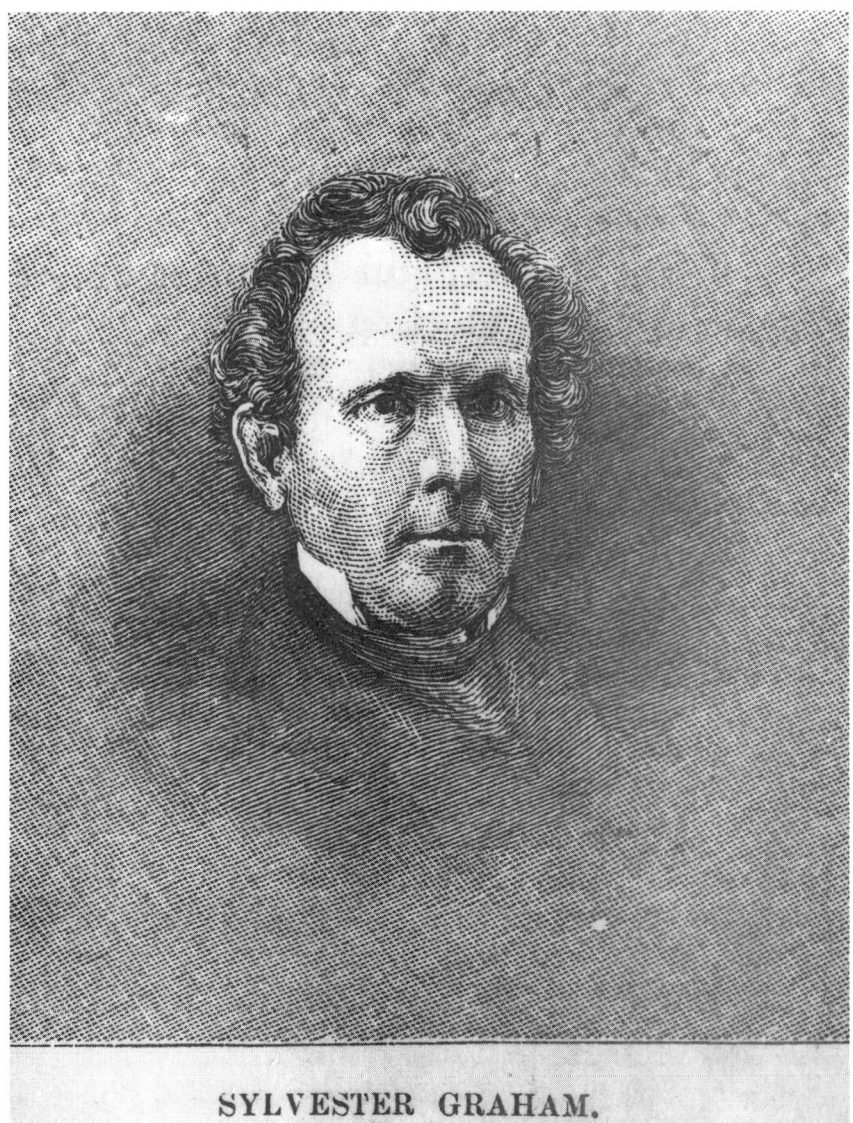

Sylvester Graham, an American preacher and vegetarian from the 1800s, believed that high-fiber, natural food could cure disease and other digestive ills. He is famous as the namesake of the graham cracker. [Courtesy of the Library of Congress]

The 1960s were also a time of sweeping social change and rebellion against authority. Small pockets of Americans linked pacifism and vegetarianism as ways to protest our country's policies, especially its involvement in the Vietnam War. An increasing number of U.S. vegetarians embraced authors such as Frances Moore Lappé, who criticized the typical American diet in her 1971 book, *Diet for a Small Planet*. Lappé called cattle "reverse protein factories" that consumed more food than they provided as meat. She suggested that America's large-scale, industrialized food production damaged the environment. She rejected factory farming methods, the use of antibiotics, and the cruelty inflicted upon livestock.

Lappé called for a worldwide change to a vegetarian diet, telling readers it had global implications for the environment and for future generations: "What we eat is within our control, yet the act ties us to the economic, political and ecological order of the whole planet. Even an apparently small change, consciously choosing a diet that is good for both our bodies and for the earth, can lead to a series of choices that transform our whole lives."[5] Lappé joined Joseph Collins to found the Institute for Food and Development Policy, commonly known as Food First, an organization that continues to support local food production and alternatives to corporate agriculture.

In their book *Food First: Beyond the Myth of Scarcity* (1977), Lappé and Collins claimed that starvation and hunger were not due to insufficient food supplies, but were caused by government and corporate policies designed to keep food from reaching those who needed it most. Aspects of that argument remain in the public debate. Fast-forward to May 2008, when an issue of *U.S. News and World Report* linked unequal food distribution and American waste to the current global food shortage. The article reported that some 25,000 people die each day of hunger in countries around the world, while U.S. consumers annually throw away 96 billion pounds of food—an average of 320 pounds of food per person.[6]

Diet for a Small Planet sold in excess of three million copies, and over the years influenced and encouraged other advocates of modern vegetarianism, such as the animal rights organization People for the Ethical Treatment of Animals (PETA). Formed in 1980, PETA embraced the idea of vegetarianism for humane reasons and attacked a variety of targets from chicken farms to fast-food restaurants. They published horror stories and photographs illustrating slaughterhouse conditions, and threw paint on women wearing fur coats, all in the name of bringing public attention to the inhumanity of animal agriculture and other animal cruelty issues.

On an international scale, vegetarian and environmental activists now connect what they call damaging animal agriculture practices to global warming. In December 2007, over 30,000 protestors joined the National

Climate March in London to publicize the link between climate change and the environmental effects of corporate livestock farming and damage from factory farms. The London-based march was sponsored by PETA, the Vegan Society, the Help International Plant Protein Organization (HIPPO), and the World Health Organization (WHO).

The march highlighted environmental hazards such as the billions of tons of manure produced each year by factory farms. The manure is spread on fields and often applied in quantities too large for the soil to absorb. This causes it to run off in heavy rains, polluting nearby land and water. The Organization for Economic Cooperation and Development (OECD) lists pollution from fertilizer and manure as one of the most serious water quality issues in the United States and Europe. The OECD was established in 1961, and provides international statistics and economic data while it compiles trade, environment, agriculture, and technology trends in some 30 nations.

The Diet and Health Connection

Studies by mainstream organizations from the WHO to the ADA and the American Cancer Society confirm that a vegetarian diet can improve health. A recent report by the American Institute on Cancer Research (AICR) and the World Cancer Research Fund (WCRF), released in November 2007, showed a link between colon cancer and processed meats such as hot dogs and salami—a link they suggested was as strong as the connection between lung cancer and cigarettes. The AICR report was based on five years of analysis by teams of independent researchers, international experts, and peer reviewers who examined more than 7,000 health studies.

The AICR recommendations for cancer prevention were clear: "Eat more of a variety of vegetables, fruits, whole grains and legumes such as beans," and "Limit consumption of red meats (such as beef, pork, and lamb) and avoid processed meats."[7] In fact, medical costs linked to eating meat are estimated to be $30 billion to $60 billion per year, based upon the higher prevalence of cancer as well as obesity, hypertension, heart disease, diabetes, gallstones, and foodborne illnesses among meat eaters when compared with vegetarians.[8] The American Cancer Society (ACS) released its own recommendation, suggesting that a diet high in vegetables and fruits and low in animal fat and meat provides a reduced risk of some of the most common cancers. The society's guidelines for cancer prevention include a similar recommendation to eat a diet "with an emphasis on plant sources."[9]

Some high-profile researchers also publicly support vegetarianism. A landmark study of diet habits conducted in China and designed by Dr. T. Colin Campbell, a nutritional biochemist at Cornell University, demonstrated how diets protect against cancer and other degenerative diseases. Campbell's project, known as the China Study, gathered statistics and information to illustrate the complex relationship between nutrition, lifestyle factors, diet, and degenerative diseases. Researchers collected data during the 1980s from some 6,500 rural Chinese who ate only local foods. Campbell ultimately concluded that a vast majority of all cancers, cardiovascular diseases, and other chronic illnesses can be prevented by a plant-based diet. But Campbell complained that American doctors are reluctant to suggest a meatless diet to their patients. "If we are reasonably sure of what our data from these studies are telling us, then why must we be reticent about recommending a diet which we know is safe and healthy? I personally have great faith in the public. We must tell them that a diet of roots, stems, seeds, flowers, fruit and leaves is the healthiest diet and the only diet we can promote, endorse and recommend."[10]

The well-known pediatrician Dr. Benjamin Spock promoted a vegetarian diet for children in the seventh edition of his book, *Baby and Child Care*. Spock recommended that parents stop giving dairy products to any child over the age of two. He wrote, "The process of gradual blocking of the coronary arteries begins not in adulthood, but in childhood, and the main cause of this arteriosclerosis is the steadily increasing amount of fat in the American diet, particularly saturated animal fats such as those found in meat, chicken, milk and cheeses."[11] Spock adopted a vegetarian diet in 1991. He died in 1998 at age 94; according to his wife, after he stopped eating meat and implemented a vegetarian diet, he lost 50 pounds and his health improved dramatically.

MORE REASONS TO GO VEG

Although the search for a healthy lifestyle is a big reason to turn to a vegetarian diet, some Americans are moved to vegetarianism to prevent the suffering of cows, chickens, and pigs. Thanks to PETA and other organizations, this is one of the most emotional arguments between livestock producers and animal rights advocates. Those advocates criticize a system of livestock production they say produces torture, misery, and suffering for animals. They suggest that the problem with the treatment of animals in factory farming isn't a matter of good versus evil; instead, it is a system that only recognizes animal suffering when it reduces profitability. Activists recommend a European approach to livestock production using humane methods with proven consumer support. For example, a majority of European supermarkets carry free-range eggs from hens able to walk outside. In Europe, the sale of those eggs has surpassed sales figures from caged or conventionally raised chicken eggs.[12]

Critics of PETA claim that people are higher up the food chain, which gives humans the right to produce cheap and plentiful meat. They suggest that society should focus on fixing problems with disease or crime rather waste time worrying about animals and their feelings. However, both sides agree that livestock production is big business, and business responds to consumer demand. Animal rights activists argue that it is time to end the cruel treatment of livestock. It appears that our European counterparts support the idea that U.S. conditions are cruel and unnecessary. One example is the ruling by a British judge against McDonald's in the 1997 "McLibel" case. The judge sided with two environmental activists being sued by the corporate giant. He agreed that the defendants were not guilty of libel, and were simply telling the truth about the company's cruel chicken-raising practices.

American broiler chickens are raised following guidelines issued by the National Chicken Council (NCC), a trade association for U.S. chicken growers. The NCC guidelines specify that each broiler chicken gets a space the size of a sheet of typing paper, or 96 square inches, a figure calculated to produce the greatest return on the investment by minimizing the space given to each bird.[13] Routinely, broiler chickens spend six weeks in these extremely cramped conditions, where they cannot move or turn around. When ready for market, they are packed into crates and trucked to slaughterhouses, often going for days without water. Speed is of the essence in processing the birds, and slaughterhouses are paid by the number of pounds of chickens processed each day. When they arrive at the slaughterhouse, the terrified birds are hung upside down, attached to a conveyor belt, and dipped into an electrified water bath called "the stunner." Although most are unconscious after this stage, some are not.

At the next stage, a machine slits their throats. Equipment routinely malfunctions due to the speed at which it operates, and some chickens are not killed outright during this stage. As the conveyor belt continues, the birds are plunged into a tank of scalding water; those not dead are boiled alive. Live birds struggle to escape the boiling bath and often break their ribs or legs in that struggle. This, combined with overall conditions and the vast number of chickens produced, prompted Professor John Webster of the University of Bristol's School of Veterinary Science to describe industrial chicken production as "in both magnitude and severity, the single most severe, systematic example of man's inhumanity to another sentient animal."[14]

Production guidelines for American laying hens from the United Egg Producers (UEP) suggest even less space for laying hens than for the broiler chickens—a mere 67 square inches per bird in bare wire cages, which are sometimes stacked three and four tiers high. The European Union has phased out the use of these tiny battery cages for laying hens, insisting that the birds must have a place to perch, litter to scratch in, a nesting box for laying their eggs, and about twice the space U.S. hens are given. Yet tens of thousands of U.S. hens are kept in cages, which are stacked in warehouse-sized buildings flooded with artificial light to mimic the longest days of summer and thus induce the hens to produce the maximum number of eggs all year round. The UEP program also allows American egg producers to burn off part of the chickens' beaks to prevent the birds from pecking each other while living in such crowded conditions.

Critics say that large-scale pig production conditions and related environmental problems are even more acute than those caused by intensive chicken operations. In 1975, there were more than 660,000 pig farms in the United States, producing approximately 69 million pigs a year. Over the next three decades, nearly 90 percent of those farms disappeared. By 2004, there were only 69,000 pig farms, but these produce 103 million pigs a year.[15] This boom centralizes huge amounts of pig waste, and prompted the American Public Health Association to pass a resolution in 2003 urging government officials to adopt a moratorium on the construction of new mammoth livestock factory farms.

The pigs are raised entirely indoors in crowded pens of concrete and steel, with the breeding sows kept in gestation crates or stalls a foot or so bigger than their bodies but too narrow for them to turn around. There is no straw or other bedding material, and waste passes through an opening into shallow pits. The pigs' tails are cut off to keep them from being bitten or chewed, which scientists say is a common stress reaction from intelligent animals with nothing to do but stand or lie down all day. The 25 countries of the European Union outlawed sow crates, and, based on recommendations from the EU scientific veterinary committee, all EU pigs get straw or other materials to reduce the stress of their confinement.

Animal rights activists argue that the lives of dairy cows are not much better than those of factory-farmed pigs or chickens. Although television commercials show dairy cows grazing on acres of rolling green pasture, most U.S. milk cows are confined to a single space called a "tie-stall" where they are fed and milked. A modern dairy cow gives more than three times the amount of milk produced just a few decades ago thanks to bovine somatotrophin (BST), a genetically engineered growth hormone injected into U.S. cows to boost their milk production. BST is banned in Canada and in the European Union due to concerns about its effects on people.

These U.S. dairy cows used to produce 15 to 21 pounds of milk a day and lived mostly disease-free for about 14 years when they were pasture-raised and dairy operations were smaller. Today's milk cows pump out anywhere from 90 to 120 pounds of milk a day. Statistics show that the stress from that increased production cuts their useful life span to just three or four years, and increases their rates of disease and sickness, which brings with it the increased use of antibiotics.

Vegetarians point to the use of antibiotics and steroids as a big problem, especially with U.S. dairy cows and beef cattle. Cows have a digestive system designed to eat and digest grass. Eating feed made from soybeans and corn makes cattle grow fatter quickly, but it gives them a bad case of indigestion. To offset the possibility of bacteria and illness from their feed, U.S. cattle get a diet of additives. The largest feedlot in the United States, located in Nebraska, has approximately 85,000 cattle, and the animals stand shoulder to shoulder, day after day, in their own feces. Cattle reach market weight in 14 months; during that time, because of their crowded living conditions, they are given antibiotics, along with a synthetic hormone similar to testosterone—a practice banned in Europe due to concerns about the risk of drug residues in the meat. Feed for American cattle also differs from its European counterpart in another significant way: it contains beef blood and fat as well as gelatin, chicken and pig meat, and chicken feed. The chicken feed is made up of fecal matter, dead birds, feathers, and spilled feed with beef and bone meal.

Following the mid-1980s British outbreak of mad cow disease, otherwise known as bovine spongiform encephalopathy (BSE), most countries issued total restrictions against feed containing any animal parts. The United States is the exception to the rule, and this lack of feed restriction sparked riots in South Korea in June 2008, when thousands of Koreans marched in the streets to protest government plans to allow U.S. beef imports. South Korea originally banned imports of American meat in 2003 after the first case of mad cow disease was confirmed in America. The new agreement between the United States and South Korea opened the door to imports of U.S. beef from cattle younger than 30 months;

scientists suggest that young cattle may be less susceptible to mad cow disease. Major Korean supermarkets announced that they would not sell U.S. beef, citing concerns about mad cow disease as well as other safety issues following the February 2008 recall of beef from a California based-slaughterhouse—the largest beef recall in U.S. history.

OTHER REASONS TO AVOID MEAT

Until the United States stops allowing animal parts in cattle feed, other countries will continue to reject American beef imports due to fears about transmissible spongiform encephalopathy, a fatal disease that takes decades to show symptoms in humans. Animal rights activists and vegetarians say mad cow disease is just one of many potential risks from meat already silently harming Americans. The Environmental Protection Agency (EPA) estimates that consumers ingest measurable residues of pesticides and other toxic chemicals with meat, fish, and dairy products. Fish have been found to contain PCBs and heavy metals such as mercury or lead, while meat and dairy products are laced with steroids, hormones, antibiotics, and arsenic.

It is standard practice for U.S. poultry growers to add arsenic to chicken feed; the additive is banned in Europe. At least 70 percent of young chickens raised in the United States get arsenic in their feed at some point during their six-week lifespan.[16] Although some human exposure to arsenic is directly related to its natural occurrence, arsenic feed additives leave measurable levels of arsenic in raw chicken. Vegetarians point to studies showing that various forms of arsenic can cause cancer even at low levels, and can contribute to other diseases including heart disease, diabetes, and even declines in intellectual ability.

USDA scientists, writing in the 2004 *Environmental Health Perspectives,* a journal of the National Institutes of Health, found measurable levels of arsenic in young chickens as well as in other meat and poultry products. A 2006 independent study by the Institute for Agriculture and Trade Policy (IATP) followed up on those findings. The study detected arsenic in 55 percent of the uncooked supermarket chicken products tested, and in 100 percent of fast-food chicken products tested.[17] The IATP was founded in 1986 to support healthy global food and agriculture policies and to stop the increasing loss of small farms.

U.S. consumers may wonder whether the benefits of arsenic in chicken feed outweigh the risks, especially given that the arsenic and other additives are not used to treat sickness. According to industry officials, in order to produce more animals in less time and at a lower price, chicken producers put antibiotics, arsenic, and other additives in chicken feed as a precaution. This practice increases exposure to arsenic and antibiotics for Americans, because consumers are eating more chicken than ever before. Figures from the IATP in 2004 showed a 65 percent increase in the production of U.S. broiler chickens over the previous 14 years. Annual chicken consumption is up by 253 percent over the same period, from over 32 pounds per person yearly to a whopping 81 pounds per person.[18]

Officials with the National Chicken Council defend the use of arsenic, and argue that the arsenic in chicken feed is organic, not the toxic inorganic form. The IATP disagrees, and has reported that some organic arsenic appears to be transformed within the chicken into inorganic arsenic. Even the Environmental Protection Agency (EPA) estimates that 65 percent of arsenic in chicken meat is inorganic arsenic.[19] At least one major U.S. chicken producer, Tyson, announced in 2006 that it was abandoning arsenic additives.

To reassure consumers about added arsenic, poultry industry officials point to the USDA Food Safety Inspection Service (FSIS), which enforces legal standards for chemical residues in food and sets "safe" levels for arsenic. In that context, it is important to remember that a "safe" level does not require that food be free of contaminants; rather, it is an acceptable amount of contamination that can be eaten or ingested without causing immediate, measurable illness. The assessment of safe levels does not consider accumulated amounts of arsenic or effects over time. Moreover, studies done on the effects of arsenic exposure routinely examine these effects in isolation, rather than in combination with the effects of other sources of contamination or of other toxic chemicals to which a person may be exposed. Americans may be getting additional arsenic exposure from contaminated drinking water, from eating plants grown in soil contaminated years ago by arsenic-laced pesticides, or from decks and playground equipment treated with arsenic preservatives. The EPA stopped the manufacture and sale of arsenic-treated lumber in 2004. At that time, more than 90 percent of all outdoor wood decks, playground sets, and other wooden structures in the United States were made of arsenic-treated wood.[20] Many of those structures are still in use today.

Another contaminant in meat creating problems for consumers was discovered by scientists at the Johns Hopkins Bloomberg School of Public Health. Researchers there conducted studies that found that chicken flesh is often contaminated with antibiotic-resistant bacteria. The FDA approved the use of antibiotics in poultry for controlling *E. coli* and other infectious organisms in 1995. By October 2000, the FDA's Center for Veterinary Medicine announced that it intended to withdraw approval for antibiotic use in poultry production because "new evidence had shown that it may not be safe for human health."[21] In 2002, two major U.S. producers, Tyson and Perdue, separately announced that they would stop using antibiotics to treat poultry flocks.

The Johns Hopkins study noted that antibiotic-free brands of chicken were not contaminated with *Campylobacter, Salmonella,* or *E. coli* bacteria. The authors compared their findings with the results from an Australian study, and discovered strong evidence to support the connection between giving chickens antibiotics and increased rates of contamination with antibiotic-resistant strains of *Campylobacter* and *Salmonella.* Australia prohibits antibiotics in poultry production.

Consumer Reports magazine conducted its own survey to determine whether U.S. chicken contained measurable amounts of antibiotic-resistant bacteria. The investigation found that over 83 percent of fresh, whole chickens bought nationwide tested positive for *Campylobacter* or *Salmonella,* the leading bacterial causes of foodborne disease in this country.[22] The investigation also tested the bacteria from the chickens for sensitivity to antibiotics, and found that there was resistance to individual drugs as well as to whole classes of drugs. These results suggest that people sickened by bacteria from chicken may discover that certain antibiotics will not work in treating their illness, and chicken treated with antibiotics tend to have more bacterial contamination.

Salmonella and *Campylobacter* bacteria cause varying degrees of intestinal illness depending on age, immune system health, and other factors. The effects of *Salmonella* range from mild flu-like symptoms to organ failure and death, depending on the severity of the infection and the immune health of the person infected. *Campylobacter* can lead to meningitis, arthritis, and Guillain-Barré syndrome, a neurological disorder. *Consumer Reports* cited the experience of a 40-year-old Indiana man who suspected he was infected with *Campylobacter* from undercooked chicken strips he ate at a Phoenix restaurant while on vacation in 2002. Days after his symptoms appeared, he lost feeling in his feet and legs. He was eventually diagnosed with Guillain-Barré syndrome. He continues to have problems walking, and his lawsuit was settled out of court in April 2006 without admission of liability.

REASONS TO EAT MEAT

Globally, meat remains a popular food for people who are able to afford it. Newly affluent families from China to Brazil doubled their meat consumption in the last two decades. In the United States, per capita consumption is more than four and a half pounds a week, and overall U.S. meat consumption has nearly quadrupled since 1950.[23] Meat eaters may wonder whether meatless meals will supply the protein, vitamins, minerals, or energy they need. Those worries were supported by a May 2000 article in the *Journal of the American Dietetic Association,* which described a study of overweight and obese men and how diet affected their ability to improve their health through resistance training. Some of the men in the study ate a beef-based diet; others followed a lacto-ovo-vegetarian eating plan. The men who ate meat showed an improved response to the resistance training over those who ate vegetarian meals.

Meat eaters suggest that, by making thoughtful choices, they can enjoy a diet relatively low in fat compared to vegetarians who eat whole dairy products such as cheese, milk, cream, and butter. The National Pork Producers Council Web site noted that pork today is lower in fat, calories, and cholesterol than it was decades ago. The National Cattlemen's Beef Association (NCBA) touts the benefits of beef on its Web site. A study commissioned by the NCBA reported that people who routinely eat beef easily meet their daily intake levels for iron, zinc, protein, and some B vitamins.

Eating meat eliminates worry about vitamin B12 deficiencies. This vitamin is essential to the function of the brain, spinal cord, and nerves, and helps maintain the protective coverings around nerve fibers. Although a deficiency is rare, early symptoms include fatigue and weakness. If left for too long, symptoms can escalate to shortness of breath, heart palpitations, and nerve damage.

The ability to absorb vitamin B12 differs from person to person, and because it is conserved within our bodies, our daily requirement is miniscule. Although recommended intake levels differ based on age and other factors including pregnancy, the Daily Recommended Intake for those above the age of 13 is 2.4 micrograms (mcg) per day. Nonvegetarians get their B12 from animal products. Vegetarians and vegans can, however, get B12 from fortified foods and vitamin supplements, as well as from fermented foods such as miso, tempeh, tamari, sauerkraut, spirulina, and algae.

Pro-meat organizations are not afraid to take on critics such as PETA or other animal activists. The Center for Consumer Freedom (CCF), the beef, poultry, and pork associations, and other industry groups say that they support a vegetarian diet for the small percentage of people who enjoy it. But the CCF, a nonprofit coalition supported by restaurants, food companies, and consumers, openly criticizes any large-scale adoption of vegetarian eating. The center's Web site challenges what it calls the rising wave of anti-agribusiness activism that threatens the U.S. food and beverage industry.

Basic Vegetarian Nutrition

Good nutrition for vegetarians and vegans is not difficult to achieve. Basically, nutrients are divided into five groups: proteins, carbohydrates, fats, vitamins, and minerals. A meatless diet does not automatically lead to protein deficiency. Remember, it wasn't until the twentieth century that meat was a common protein source. When Lappé addressed "where to get your protein" in her 1971 book, she described a process called protein complementing. This was a way for a vegetarian to combine a low-protein food, lacking certain amino acids, with foods high in those nutrients. Rice and beans are a good example of protein complementing; when eaten together, the rice and beans compliment their individual deficiencies. Today, research has shown that protein complementing isn't necessary. Nutritionists say the human body is efficient enough to absorb the essential amino acids from a well-balanced diet whether the foods are combined or not, especially because every food, with the exception of sugar, fat, and fruit, has some protein in it.

Proteins

People require some 20 amino acids for optimum health; 11 of those are manufactured by our bodies, but the other 9 must come from the foods we eat. All the required amino acids can come from plant foods or can be manufactured by the human body. People need protein to maintain healthy skin, bones, muscles, and organs. Many plant foods, such as soy, are protein-rich and also provide protective phytochemicals. Beans, peas, and lentils are richer in magnesium and lower in sulfur amino acids than meat, which means they cause the body to excrete less calcium. Legumes provide iron, zinc, a number of B vitamins, and lots of fiber.

Where can the average American go to find out what constitutes appropriate nutrient levels of vitamins, minerals, carbohydrates, proteins, and fats? The Recommended Dietary Allowance (RDA) was established by the USDA to provide nutrition guidelines for Americans. Recently, the RDA was replaced by the Dietary Reference Intake (DRI), which includes four different reference values and offers more flexible numbers based on activity level, age, and other factors. According to the USDA, the DRI for protein is 0.8 grams of protein per kilogram of body weight (g/kg)—about 45 grams for an average woman and 55 grams for an average man. This includes a margin to account for individual variations, and applies to vegetarians and meat-eaters alike. Recommended intake levels during pregnancy, lactation and infancy through adolescence differ slightly.

Although some protein is necessary, high intakes of protein can be harmful—particularly animal protein, which studies show can contribute to

VEGETARIANS

heart disease, stroke, and colorectal cancer. Animal proteins are associated with cholesterol and saturated fat, whereas plant foods are cholesterol-free and most are low in saturated fat. The protein in common vegetarian foods ranges from 18 grams of protein in one cup of cooked lentils or black, navy, kidney, or pinto beans to 28 grams of protein in one cup of cooked soybeans. In comparison, a fast-food hamburger patty made of a quarter pound of beef has 19 grams of protein, and a chicken leg has 15 grams.

Carbohydrates

There are three types of carbohydrates: monosaccharides, or simple sugars; disaccharides, composed of two monosaccharides; and polysaccharides, also known as complex carbohydrates or starches. Carbohydrates are an important source of energy for the brain, central nervous system, and muscle cells. They are found in sugars, fruits, vegetables, cereals, and grains. Carbohydrates are also broken down into two other categories on nutrition labels: fiber and sugar. The simple sugars provide energy but lack fiber, vitamins, or minerals. The complex carbohydrates or starches contain lots of fiber, vitamins and minerals and are naturally low in fat. Many types of grains are good sources of complex carbohydrates, and whole grains such as brown rice and whole wheat provide particularly rich nutrients and fiber.

All carbohydrates are eventually broken down into sugars in the body. The difference between complex carbohydrates and simple sugars is that complex carbohydrates are broken down gradually and provide energy over a longer period of time. The fiber in these foods is important. Fiber provides health benefits by preventing constipation as well as lowering the risk of diabetes and heart disease. But all carbohydrates are not created equal. Nutritionists caution that the monosaccharides, or simple sugars, present a nutritional problem on two fronts. First, filling up on high-sugar foods such as soft drinks, cookies, sweets, and fruit drinks can contribute to weight gain. Second, simple-sugar foods contain very few vitamins or minerals and can lead to poor health if they are continuously eaten instead of more nutritious foods. Someone with a diet of 2,000 calories per day should eat about 300 grams of carbohydrates. A slice of whole wheat bread has 20 grams of carbohydrates, a medium baked potato has some 51 grams, an apple has 21 grams, and a tablespoon of sugar about 12 grams.

Fats

Despite their poor image, fats aren't all bad. Some fat is needed to supply energy and help the body absorb the fat-soluble vitamins, A, D, E, and

K. Fats contain saturated or unsaturated fatty acids, two of which—linoleic and linolenic acid—are essential and must be provided in the diet. Luckily, both those fatty acids are widely found in plant foods. When choosing fats, the best options for vegetarians and meat eaters alike are the monounsaturated and polyunsaturated fats, which can lower the risk of heart disease by reducing cholesterol levels.

Monounsaturated fats include olive, canola, and peanut oils, and can be found in avocados and most nuts. Polyunsaturated fats come from safflower, corn, sunflower, soy, cottonseed, and vegetable oils. Unlike monounsaturated fats, which begin to solidify when chilled, polyunsaturated fats remain liquid whether at room temperature or in the refrigerator. The polyunsaturated fats called omega-3 fatty acids are especially beneficial, and can be found in flaxseeds, flax oil, and walnuts and, in small amounts, in soybean and canola oils.

Saturated fats come from red meat, poultry, butter, and whole milk as well as coconut, palm, and other tropical oils. These fats are also high in cholesterol, and although dietary cholesterol isn't technically a fat, it is known to increase blood cholesterol levels, as does saturated fat. The human body produces cholesterol during the process of cell building, and cholesterol can leave behind fatty deposits or plaques in arteries. When the plaques build up, they reduce blood flow and increase the risk of a heart attack or stroke.

Along with saturated fats, trans fat can add a big dose of unhealthy fat to the standard American diet. Trans fat, also known as trans-fatty acid, is made by adding hydrogen to vegetable oil during a process called hydrogenation. This keeps the fat from turning rancid and increases the shelf life of items. Trans fat is commonly found in margarine, in commercial baked goods such as cookies and cakes, and in fried foods such as doughnuts. Scientists now believe that, gram for gram, trans fats are twice as damaging as saturated fat. In January 2006, food manufacturers became required to include trans fat content on nutrition labels.

The U.S. Surgeon General, the National Academy of Sciences, the American Heart Association, the American Dietetic Association, the USDA, and the U.S. Department of Health and Human Services (HHS) all recommend keeping dietary fat intake at 30 percent or less of total calories. Fat is measured in grams, so for someone eating a diet of 2,000 calories per day, daily fat intake should be 65 grams or less, preferably coming from monounsaturated or polyunsaturated sources. The 2005 *Dietary Guidelines for Americans* also strongly recommends consuming less than

10 percent of daily calories from saturated fats and keeping trans fat consumption as low as possible.

Vitamins

Vitamins are a key area where many Americans fall nutritionally short, and vegetarians—who eat a rainbow of fruits and vegetables rich in vitamins, minerals, and fiber—have a nutritional advantage. Vitamin A, or beta carotene, can be found in yellow, red, or orange vegetables such as carrots and tomatoes, fruits such as apricots and peaches, and leafy green vegetables. B vitamins are important for the health of the nervous system and play a role in the metabolism of carbohydrates, fats, and proteins. B vitamins are water-soluble and are not stored in the body, so they need to be supplied daily by a healthy diet. Good sources of B vitamins, except for B12, include whole grain cereals, wheat germ, nuts, seeds, yeasts, and green vegetables.

Vitamin B12 deficiencies are rare. The vitamin is found in meat, dairy, and eggs, so vegetarians and vegans need to monitor their intake to make sure they get enough. Many veggie burgers, soy products, and breakfast cereals are fortified with B12. Even though little is needed, B12 plays important roles in the production of DNA and RNA, in making red blood cells, and in keeping the nervous system operating.

Fruits, especially citrus fruits such as oranges and lemons, are great sources of vitamin C, also known as ascorbic acid. Vegetables including broccoli, potatoes, and tomatoes contain vitamin C, as do strawberries, kiwifruit, and cantaloupe. Vitamin C helps to fight disease and infection, aids the repair of tissue, and acts as an antioxidant. The recommended amount of vitamin C for healthy people is 60 mg per day. Taking extra vitamin C as treatment for a cold is a common practice; however, research on the benefits of these megadoses remains inconclusive.

Healthy bones depend on calcium, but calcium needs vitamin D to be absorbed into the body. Vitamin D is also important for building and maintaining muscles. Known as the sunshine vitamin, vitamin D is made in the body when sunlight hits the skin. So 15 minutes or less of sunshine three times a week can provide enough of the vitamin for a healthy adult. Vitamin D is also found in fortified soy beverages, orange juice, and cereals.

The term vitamin E describes a family of eight antioxidants—alpha, beta, gamma, and delta tocopherol, and alpha, beta, gamma and delta tocotrienol. Alpha-tocopherol (α-tocopherol) is the most active form in the human body, and is the form of vitamin E found in the largest quantities in the blood and tissue. Because vitamin E is fat-soluble, it is generally found in rich foods such as avocado, nuts, olives, and vegetable oils, and also in spinach and other green leafy vegetables. The results of studies on the use of vitamin E in the treatment and prevention of several diseases, particularly in cancer and heart disease, are still inconclusive.

Vitamin K is known as the clotting vitamin; without it blood would not clot. This fat-soluble vitamin is stored in fatty tissue and is found in spinach and other green leafy vegetables, cabbage, cauliflower, soybeans, and cereals. It is also made by the bacteria that line the gastrointestinal tract. Vitamin K deficiency is very rare.

Minerals

Of all the minerals in the human body, calcium warrants the most attention, because it is the most abundant. 98 percent of it is found in the bones and teeth. Bones are living systems, and when the body is at rest, calcium is pulled from the bones to be used elsewhere. Calcium also plays a role in the proper functioning of the heart, muscles, and nerves that maintain blood flow. Although requirements for calcium vary depending on age and other factors, an average adult should take in between 1,000 and 1,300 milligrams (mg) per day. The body absorbs calcium more efficiently when small amounts are eaten throughout the day, and calcium absorption is another important factor in good health. Studies show that excess protein in the diet causes a loss of calcium, which may be a factor in the growing incidence of osteoporosis in the United States. Although it is important to get enough calcium, more is not always better, because high intakes of calcium interfere with the absorption of iron, zinc, and manganese. Good vegetarian sources of dietary calcium include tofu, dried peas and beans, collard greens, broccoli, kale, and calcium-fortified foods such as orange juice and cereals.

Iron is a trace mineral necessary for oxygen transport and storage, energy metabolism, and DNA synthesis. Although most people associate iron with animal foods such as red meat, liver and fish, iron can also be found in spinach and chard; molasses; dried fruits such as prunes, apricots, and raisins; and whole grains. Quinoa and amaranth contain about four to six times more iron than other grains. Low iron levels can cause anemia, so women often need iron supplements, especially in their teens and child-bearing years when iron is lost through blood. On the other hand, excess iron can accumulate in the body to toxic levels, so iron supplements should only be prescribed by a doctor.

Chromium is a trace element important in producing a substance called glucose tolerance factor (GTF), a compound that works with insulin to move glucose into cells where it can be used to produce energy. A diet filled with processed foods depletes chromium, which is used in the metabolism of sugary foods. Copper also plays a role in the body's energy production, as well as in iron metabolism, brain and nervous system function, and the formation of connective tissue. Zinc is important in reproduction and, like copper, in neurological function. In addition, nearly one hundred enzymes are dependent on zinc for their function. Zinc comes from the soil where plants are grown, but some fertilizers make it hard for plants to absorb zinc from the ground. Grains are a good source of zinc, and quinoa and amaranth provide a higher level of zinc than other grains. Copper and zinc have similar properties and provide a balancing effect on each other.

Another trace mineral is selenium, a natural antioxidant that assists the immune system, protects against cancer, and is a factor in fertility. The richest plant source for selenium is the Brazil nut, a single nut contains double the daily requirement of 50 micrograms (mcg). Other rich sources are nuts, seeds, and grains. High doses of selenium are toxic, and no more than 300 mcg a day are recommended.

The mineral manganese serves as an antioxidant, and protects cells and assists in the formation of healthy bones and cartilage. Whole grains are good sources. Magnesium is necessary in a host of essential metabolic reactions from energy production to the synthesis of DNA. In some cases it has improved vision in glaucoma patients and been shown to reduce hyperactivity in children with low magnesium levels. Whole grains are an important source, but, unfortunately, magnesium has been refined out of many of today's processed foods.

Potassium is essential to every cell in the human body and works in tandem with sodium. Together, they regulate water balance in the body, and their equilibrium also stimulates nerve impulses for the heart and other muscle contractions. The typical American diet of processed and convenience foods may contain insufficient potassium as well as an excess of sodium. That imbalance can lead to high blood pressure and kidney and heart disease. Good sources of potassium include bananas, avocados, potatoes, and whole grains. Unfortunately, refined grains have the two most nutrition-filled parts, the bran and germ, removed. Vegetarians seldom have difficulty meeting their daily potassium requirement.

CAMOUFLAGING EATING DISORDERS?

The USDA Food Guide Pyramid suggests a healthy diet based on a variety of fruits, vegetables, and grains and a modest amount of healthy fat and protein. Statistics show that only one in four Americans meets these recommended intakes, and, not surprisingly, many teens eat even less. One disturbing pattern of poor nutrition involves teens with eating disorders. Recent studies have sought to measure the number of teens who hide their eating disorders behind the healthy façade of vegetarianism. The National Association of Anorexia and Associated Disorders estimates that more than 8 million Americans suffer from full-blown eating disorders, and a small number may try to hide their symptoms by changing to a vegetarian diet. However, data suggest that teens who adopt a vegetarian diet do not automatically end up with an eating disorder.

It is important for parents and doctors to make a distinction between teens who choose to be vegetarians to maintain good health and those who use vegetarianism as an excuse to avoid eating. The two most common eating disorders in the United States are anorexia nervosa and bulimia, or bingeing and purging. Excessive dieting, binge eating, intentional vomiting, and laxative abuse are among signs associated with these eating disorders; they are more common in girls than in boys, although figures for young men are rising.

Is Vegetarianism for You?

The word "vegetarian" comes from the Latin word *vegetus*, which means strength. The days of the skinny, granola-eating, tofu-loving vegetarians are passed. Today's meatless eaters are normal, robust, average Americans who wish to improve their health and their impact on the environment. Still, vegetarianism isn't a miracle cure for poor eating habits or bad food choices. Variety is fundamental whether you eat meat or not. Nutritionists say the biggest mistake new vegetarians make is to fill up on fattening foods such as cheese, French fries, pizza, and pasta. The best diet for everyone is rich in fiber and complex carbohydrates, low in fat, and full of fresh vegetables and fruits. Vegetarianism has many merits and many new supporters. Although Americans love to eat meat, it is clear that good health is tied to lowering one's intake of saturated fats. Moreover, if food prices continue to soar, then American wallets and waistlines may reap even more benefits from meatless meals.

CHAPTER 8

Organic Food: Better or Just More Expensive?

Organics are the new darling of the food industry. More than a niche market, they have expanded during the past decade by a healthy 20 percent annually, while other industries struggle to stay afloat. Organic food and beverage sales topped $17 billion dollars in 2006, up from $1 billion in 1990 according to U.S. Department of Agriculture (USDA) figures.[1] Everyone from Trader Joe's and Whole Foods to Wal-Mart and the big-box supermarkets are rushing to fill their shelves, produce bins, and meat counters with anything and everything organic.

As the small and large organic producers jockey to get their products to consumers, the big corporations new to organics are working to change the stringent organic rules to avoid the higher costs that come from having to meet such exacting standards. This leaves small-scale organic farmers struggling to keep their customers in the face of rising food prices and fierce competition from the big players.

In this mad dash to give consumers unprecedented organic choices, the questions remain, are organics healthier or just more expensive? And are they better for the environment, farmers, or consumers? Another major issue looming over the organic food industry is the question of scale. Does the move toward industrial-sized organic farming undermine the benefits and identity of organic food itself? Or is it a logical way to introduce more consumers to organics? That red hot debate between "little organics" and "big organics" is a factor in purchasing decisions for some Americans. To sort out the issues and the players, it's necessary to examine the organics of today along with the history of the organic movement.

HISTORY OF ORGANICS

From the earliest days, supporters of organic farming envisioned a way to feed people and build a food ecosystem using sustainable practices, working with rather than against nature. Another aim of organic agriculture was to nurture the earth and achieve a harmonious fit with the land and the local community. Organic food today remains a reaction to the use of synthetic fertilizers in industrial agriculture, which depletes the soil, pushes small farmers off the land, and replaces them with single-crop agribusiness operations.

At the beginning of the twentieth century, the British led the organic movement with people such as Sir Arthur Howard, an agronomist influenced by Eastern spiritual concepts and a belief in a connected circle of life. Howard's organic philosophy flourished when he was sent by his government to India in 1905 to establish an agricultural research base. He was immediately intrigued by the farming methods of the Indian peasants.

The local farmers fertilized with composted animal and vegetable wastes, and Howard noticed that they had excellent soil fertility, abundant crops, and livestock seemingly immune to pests and diseases. Howard theorized that the health of plants, animals, and people depended on maintaining a state of equilibrium between living creatures and the environment, a harmony of the whole system. He also decided that health was not the absence of disease, but, rather, disease was an indicator of bad management and should be used to identify mistakes and find solutions.

Howard then took his hypothesis and applied it to livestock. He exposed healthy cattle to a range of diseases, including foot and mouth disease (FMD), to study their resistance. Scientists first discovered foot and mouth disease in the sixteenth century, and the disease still threatens the cattle industry. A major epidemic of FMD occurred in the United Kingdom in 2001; to stop the spread of the disease, officials slaughtered some three million animals, 95 percent of which were perfectly healthy. That outbreak cost the UK economy an estimated 20 billion pounds and decimated rural livestock producers.[2]

Howard's cattle contracted foot and mouth disease only once in his 25-year study, during a summer drought when the cattle were fed a poor diet and still provided heavy field work. Howard noted that after the animals were rested and given better food, the FMD disappeared. Howard repeated his experiments at three different research stations with various groups of livestock, until he was convinced that FMD was linked to malnutrition.

Howard came to believe that there was a connection between increased animal diseases and the increased use of artificial fertilizers. He disagreed with the use of chemical fertilizers, first developed in the 1840s by German chemist Justus von Liebig. Von Liebig had discovered the right balance of nitrogen, potassium, and phosphorous to feed plants as a replacement for manure. He thought the organic components of manure were unnecessary, and that plant fertility improved due to the minerals in the manure. His fertilizers focused on feeding the plants rather than on improving the biological activity in the soil. Howard thought Von Liebig missed the big picture with his narrow focus. Instead, Howard considered the health of soil, plant, animal, and human a connected chain, with widespread vegetable and animal pests or diseases a weak link in the chain. Most importantly, he thought that the undernourishment of the soil was a prescription for disaster. "The failure to maintain a healthy agriculture has largely cancelled out all the advantages we have gained from our improvements in hygiene, in housing and in our medical discoveries."[3]

In 1941, Jerome Irving Rodale discovered Howard's writings just as American agriculture fully embraced chemical fertilizers; in just one year, from 1940 to 1941, U.S. fertilizer use increased sevenfold.[4] USDA figures for 2006 showed that conventional U.S. agriculture used over 21 million tons of chemical fertilizer that year. Rodale, one of the first advocates for sustainable agriculture and organic farming in the United States, was born in 1898 in New York City; like many early nutrition advocates, he was frequently ill as a child. Educated as an accountant, he briefly worked for the federal government as a tax auditor before going into business with his brother and moving to Emmaus, Pennsylvania.

After Rodale read Howard's theories, he bought a 60-acre Pennsylvania farm and began a lifetime correspondence with Howard about farming ideas and methods. He also started a publishing company and released *Organic Farming* magazine, but few farmers were interested in subscribing. Undaunted, Rodale widened the scope of the publication to include home gardeners, and in 1942 he rereleased the magazine as *Organic Farming and Gardening*. Howard served as a long-distance associate editor. Five years later, Rodale formed the Soil and Health Foundation to boost scientific research, education, teaching, and training on organic farming.

Rodale continued to promote organic farming and gardening techniques on his farm through the 1960s. The publication of Rachel Carson's book, *Silent Spring* (1962), also focused attention on organic agriculture and the environment. In 1971, the *New York Times Magazine* named

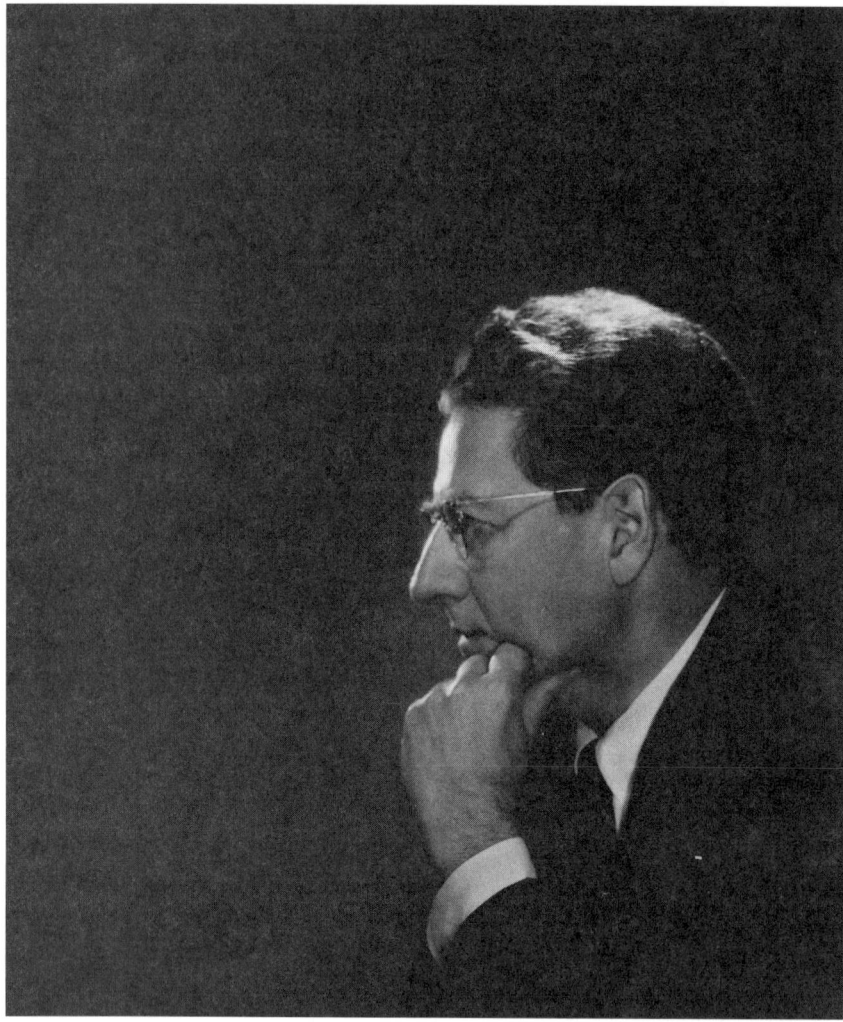

J. I. Rodale was an early American proponent of organic farming. He published the *Organic Farming and Gardening* magazine in 1942 and formed the Soil and Health Foundation, later renamed the Rodale Institute, to educate Americans about the benefits of organic farming. [Courtesy of Rodale, Inc.]

Rodale "Guru of the Organic Food Cult." His organic gospel was based on three key elements. First, the long-range health of the soil is paramount and is enhanced by a high level of organic matter. Second, organic matter offers a more balanced delivery of nutrients to plants than do chemical fertilizers. Finally, a delicate balance in the soil keeps pathogenic organisms in check, but chemical fertilizers and pesticides upset that balance.[5] According to the *New York Times Magazine* article, Rodale's stance contradicted the official USDA position on organic plants, which stated that there was no evidence that organic plants were any better than their conventionally grown counterparts. The 1970s and 1980s saw an increase in organic farming and organic produce, and the growth of the Rodale organization. The industry that began with experimental garden plots was now turning into large farms and an increasing variety of products labeled "organic."

Legislation and the USDA Designation

As early as the 1950s, a handful of American consumers started buying products grown without chemicals. Farmers experimenting with organic systems generally marketed directly to those consumers or to small health food stores. By the late 1960s, a new generation of environmentally friendly consumers demanded more and more products without chemicals, creating a need for larger natural foods supermarkets and cooperative stores. Sales of organic items continued to climb. Industry analysts estimate that retail sales of organic foods rose to some $4 billion dollars annually by the early 1990s. Even so, mainstream agriculture still considered this a specialty market, taking in just one percent of overall U.S. consumer spending on food and groceries.

In a move to support organic farmers and to verify that products were actually organic, private organizations along with nonprofit groups put together certification standards as early as the 1970s. The first organization to offer third-party organic certification formed in 1973 as the California Certified Organic Farmers. At that time, various states approached regulations differently. Today, most states still do not mandate third-party certification of organic foods. Of the states with legislation, some allow voluntary certification, whereas others demand that all organic products be certified. Some states provide their own organic certification services, and others hire private agencies.

Even with certification increasingly available from state agencies and private companies, many organic food producers and processors were not satisfied. Big differences in standards among certifying agents kept growers and consumers uncertain about the true meaning of the term "organic." Big agribusiness wanted a flexible definition to make it easier and cheaper for large corporations to get into organic production. Many were also concerned that anything not labeled organic, such as irradiated or genetically modified foods, would be considered unhealthy in the eyes of American consumers. The need to reach a consensus on certification standards and labels prompted many in the organic industry to petition Congress for assistance.

The Organic Foods Production Act (OFPA), enacted as part of the 1990 farm bill, was designed to develop a common language and consistent uniform standards for organic food. Unfortunately, as the business of organics had grown, so had the friction between small organic farmers and whole food purists on one hand, and the profit-driven large factory farms on the other. With profits and principles at stake, the OFPA set up a National Organic Standards Board (NOSB) as an advisory panel to help both sides reach a consensus.

The board was made up of 15 members appointed by the secretary of agriculture, and included farmers, retailers, scientists, certifiers, and consumers. Whereas regulations involving organic farming seemed fairly clear-cut, crafting rules for processing organic food was tougher. Both sides wanted their needs met, but neither wanted to compromise. The NOSB finished its first draft of recommendations and submitted them to the USDA in 1995. For two years, the USDA labored over the standards, and in 1997 it released a document that was a far cry from what small organic farmers expected. Bowing to pressure from agribusiness interests, the USDA standards allowed genetically modified crops, irradiated foods, and sewage sludge in "organic" food products.

The organic community bombarded the USDA with the largest recorded response to a proposed rule in recent department history; 275,000 negative comments poured into the agency.[6] At the same time, the USDA was under political pressure from Clinton administration officials working to improve U.S. exports of genetically modified foods in Europe. Politically, it made sense for USDA officials to include genetically modified organisms in the organic standards as a way to avoid undercutting administration efforts. But it made no sense to supporters of organics, and they expressed their outrage to USDA officials. Another three years passed before the USDA reissued the standards in 2000; this time genetically modified organisms, irradiation, and sewage sludge in organic production were gone.

While the debate over the meaning of the word "organic" continued, another struggle was developing between big organics—the huge agribusiness operations—and little organics, the small organic growers. The big organics corporations wanted relief from the 1990 legislation that prohibited synthetic food additives and manufacturing agents, which they claimed were vital to organic processed foods. They pressed for the standards to include a list of permissible additives and synthetics that could be substituted if the organic versions were not commercially available. The government left the decision on what it meant for a product to be "unavailable" in organic form to the interpretation of each certifying agency or organization, creating even more confusion.

After twelve years of debate and a massive amount of public comment, the National Organic Program (NOP) was finally launched in 2002 and immediately challenged. By 2003, a Georgia chicken producer persuaded his congressional representative to loosen the rules requiring organic feed for organic livestock. The congressman added a rider to a congressional spending bill that allowed livestock producers to use cheaper, nonorganic feed and still call themselves organic if the price of organic feed was more than double the cost of regular feed. Although the bill passed, the amendment was repealed a few months later after consumers and organic producers protested in overwhelming numbers.

This constant assault on the intent of the 1990 Organic Foods Production Act (OFPA) frustrated people such as organic blueberry farmer Arthur Harvey, who reacted by filing a lawsuit against the USDA and then–Secretary of Agriculture Ann Veneman. Harvey charged that the 2002 rule did not conform to the OFPA. Harvey was a no-nonsense farmer, an organic certifier, and an active member of the Maine Organic Trade Association. Although he began his lawsuit alone, he was soon joined by several friends of the court, including the Center for Food Safety, the Rural Advancement Foundation International, Beyond Pesticides, and Roseland Farm. After he lost in the lower court, Harvey appealed, and gained the support of several environmental groups including the Organic Consumers Association, Greenpeace, and the Sierra Club.

Harvey basically objected to allowing synthetic substances in processed organic food. He filed his lawsuit out of frustration with the National Organic Standards Board (NOSB) and their approval of a list of 38 synthetic ingredients for use in organic products. The board had decided that this national list would provide a safe choice when organic ingredients weren't readily available. In response, Harvey and his supporters argued that synthetics would damage the integrity of organic foods. They predicted that if any prohibited substances accidentally made the list and were put into organic foods, the industry's credibility with consumers would be destroyed. At the same time, the large organic operations made a plea for the board to allow the 38 synthetic ingredients; otherwise, they said, it would be impossible to successfully produce organic foods for national distribution.

In 2005, the U.S. Court of Appeals based in Boston ruled in favor of Harvey on three of the seven issues he had raised about inconsistencies between the 2002 standards and the 1990 OFPA. The court gave the

USDA one year to write new rules to match the law. Meanwhile, products that failed to meet those original standards had to be reformulated or relabeled within two years of the ruling.

In response, three relevant changes were made to the OFPA's amendments; the most important was a limitation on the prohibition on synthetic ingredients, introduced by amending the wording of section 6510. This change only prohibited the addition of synthetic ingredients not on the National List. The other two changes also dealt with easing restrictions on the use of synthetic materials in organic handling and production operations. The end result gave industrial organics a list of synthetic materials for use in organic production and a tool for adding more ingredients to the list. The Organic Trade Association (OTA), which represents organic producers such as Kraft Foods and Archer Daniels Midland Company, supported the changes. Smaller organic growers and producers called it an example of how conventional agribusinesses used the system to move deeper into the organic pipeline.

BIG VERSUS LITTLE ORGANICS

The changes by Congress also put pressure on small organic farmers and producers to expand or lose their customers to bigger producers who saw synthetics as an unavoidable part of their growth. To understand the difficult choices these small organic farmers faced, it is helpful to look at two organic giants and how differently they grew. Earthbound Farm represents a classic example of a little organic grower that started from scratch and blossomed into a large-scale industrial producer with over $360 million in yearly sales.[7] Earthbound started on two-and-a-half acres of California's Carmel Valley.

Myra and Drew Goodman fell into organic farming after Myra graduated from the University of California at Berkeley in 1984. The couple moved to land owned by her parents, and discovered that the back of the property was covered in raspberries. Myra did not want to spray even though the previous tenant had grown the berries conventionally. With no farming experience, these two native New Yorkers gathered information from organic farmers, local nurseries, and the library, and perused back issues of Rodale's *Organic Gardening*. Once they figured out how to grow the berries without pesticides, they set up a roadside stand and named it Earthbound Farm. When they got word that local chefs were interested in buying baby heads of lettuce, they added lettuce to their plot of land.

Their real claim to fame came out of their desire to keep some of the lettuce for themselves. They began storing plastic bags with small portions of the washed baby lettuces in the refrigerator. The convenience was unmistakable, and the Goodmans took the idea of individual bags of lettuce to natural food stores. Bagged lettuce took off, and demand quickly exceeded supply. The rest is history; the couple made arrangements with a leading lettuce grower to ship the lettuce and a new bagged salad mix to distributors and chefs in all parts of the country, from Los Angeles to New York.

Although the Goodmans weren't the first with packaged lettuce, their product was an instant hit with consumers. Their growth exploded after Costco placed an order in 1993. Contracts with Wal-Mart and other large supermarkets soon followed. The company now represents a total of 25,000 organic acres, and the Goodmans estimate that taking their acres out of conventional production has eliminated some 270,000 pounds of pesticide and 8 million pounds of chemical fertilizer that would have been applied to those fields.[8] Although Earthbound Farm represents a big environmental improvement over conventional industrial farming, critics say there is nothing sustainable about the company's conventional transportation system or its increasing use of fossil fuels. Others have suggested that Earthbound Farm grew so large that it pushed smaller farmers out of the organic lettuce market.

Now consider Organic Valley, the nation's largest farmer-owned organic cooperative. They organized some 20 years ago with just seven family farmers, motivated by the desire to practice sustainable and organic agriculture. Today, the cooperative has grown to include some 1,266 farmers in 32 states and one Canadian province, with more than $500 million in sales in 2008.[9]

Organic Valley is the nation's largest cooperative of organic dairy, meat, egg, soy, juice, and vegetable producers. But their focus is on locally food grown, produced and sold on a small scale. Rather than ship products across the country, they introduced a program to develop regional distribution through "Pastures" brands, under which milk is produced, processed, and sold locally. One major goal of the cooperative is to improve not only their carbon footprint, but also what they call their "ecological footprint"—how members impact air, water, land, biodiversity, and toxins.

The cooperative started in 1988, with the seven original farmers, as the Coulee Region Organic Produce Pool (CROPP). All wanted to continue to use sustainable, organic farming. Organic dairy was added after they developed a brand name and successfully sold their vegetables. George L. Siemon, one of the original farmers, serves as the Chief Executive Officer (CEO) but jokingly refers to himself as the "C-E-I-E-I-O." When farmers join, they invest a small percentage of their estimated annual sales in the cooperative. For their money, they become part of a nationally recognized and respected brand, and they receive profit sharing and support in areas such as production, organic certification, farm planning, feed sourcing, veterinary consultation, and energy audits. Most importantly, they practice their beliefs.

The goals of the cooperative include protecting the environment while keeping family farmers on the land, and giving consumers access to organic food produced using humane animal treatment and sustainable farming methods. Members also compete in the national market without the stress of unmanageable rapid growth. The cooperative's membership accounts for some ten percent of America's organic farmers, according to statistics listed on their Web site. These small farmers retain their individuality and are not in danger of being bought by mainstream food giants as are other organic farmers, producers, and natural food companies. Past examples of buyouts include the purchases of Boca Burger by Kraft, Power Bar by Nestle, Kashi by Kellogg, WhiteWave and Horizon by Dean Foods Company, and Ben & Jerry's by Unilever.

One illustration of how the Organic Valley cooperative stays true to goals and customers occurred in 2004, when Organic Valley ended a direct relationship with Wal-Mart. The cooperative had been one of Wal-Mart's primary suppliers of organic milk. But the retail giant needed huge quantities of organic dairy to supply its stores. This meant individual natural food markets and other smaller stores were pushed out of the supply of organic dairy. Although members of the cooperative could have raised prices due to the short supply situation, they chose loyalty to their small vendors and original customers over profits—a choice that exemplified the principles of the organic food movement.

LABELS

In the food industry, labels are a tool consumers use to gauge the value of a product. "Organic" is one of the most recognized labels in today's supermarkets, but many consumers do not realize that there are several organic designations, and some are more organic than others.

According to the USDA, all packaged or processed food using the term "100% Organic" must contain all organic ingredients. Production processes have to meet federal organic standards and be independently verified by accredited inspectors. Items labeled "USDA Organic" are subject to a less strict standard: up to five percent of their total ingredients excluding salt and water may come from nonorganic or synthetic sources. Items labeled with the phrase "Made with organic ingredients" must include at least 70 percent organic components; the remaining 30 percent must come from the USDA-approved list of additives and synthetic ingredients. Produce, fruits, and vegetables labeled organic have to be grown without synthetic pesticides and synthetic fertilizers, and cannot be genetically engineered or irradiated.

Beef or chicken labeled as organic may not come from offspring of cloned animals; must be raised on 100 percent organic feed; must never be given growth hormones, antibiotics, or other drugs; and cannot be irradiated. The label "organic seafood," however, is meaningless, because the USDA has no laws concerning seafood standards. This means fish can be labeled organic even if it contains contaminants such as mercury or polychlorinated biphenyls (PCBs). Producers of seafood are legally allowed to make organic claims as long as they don't make use of USDA or "certified organic" logos. California state law, however, prohibits the use of organic labeling on fish and other seafood until state or federal standards are formulated.

The use of "natural" or "all natural" on a label is defined by the USDA for meat and poultry to mean the meat does not contain any artificial flavorings, colors, chemical preservatives, or synthetic ingredients. These terms are often used by manufacturers who want to portray their product as healthy even though they have not met the government's specific standards for organics. "Grass-fed" on a label suggests that the livestock received a diet of natural grass, but it also applies to cattle fed grass indoors in a pen or only allowed outside for the first few months of their lives. The label "pasture-raised" refers to animals that were allowed to roam freely outdoors where they ate grasses and other plants.

Any dairy product with an organic label comes from cows that, for at least the previous 12 months, were fed 100 percent organic feed and were not given bovine growth hormone (BGH) or antibiotics. Organic eggs come from hens fed 100 percent organic feed and raised without growth hormones or antibiotics. The term "cage-free" for poultry or eggs means little, because in both cases the birds, although not confined to cages, may still live in crowded, unhealthy conditions.

The label "free-range" or "free-roaming" on eggs or chicken also suggests that the animals may have spent at least a portion of their lives outdoors. But U.S. government standards for these terms are vague; outdoor access may be available, but it does not guarantee the animals were treated any better than animals raised in conventional factory farms. In other words, if a coop door is open for five minutes a day and the birds remain packed inside, the eggs or chicken can legally be labeled free-range. Beef or chicken labels that say "no hormones administered" or "no antibiotics added" are allowed if the producers can document those claims.

Several animal rights groups have created their own labels that include terms such as "animal compassionate," "certified humane," and "free farmed." "Animal compassionate" means sheep cannot be castrated, pig's tails may not be cut off, and electric prods can be used on cattle only in emergencies. Meat that is "certified humane" means electric prods can only be used in emergencies, but sheep can be castrated in their first week of life, and tail-docking of pigs is allowed. "Free farmed" labels include the same provisions as "certified humane," and animal rights activists consider all three designations a better standard of care than conventional livestock industry practices.

BETTER OR JUST EXPENSIVE?

Organic food products routinely cost more than their conventional counterparts, which supporters say just means organic farmers get paid a fair price for their food and their labor. Ask supporters of organic food and they will tell you the extra money spent on organic products is part of a daily contribution to their health and the health of the planet. These advocates say there are hidden costs in cheap conventional foods, including the price of environmental damage from pesticides and synthetic fertilizers; waste and overuse of energy resources needed for fertilizing, harvesting, and processing food and for transporting it thousands of miles; the effects on human health from toxic residues left by arsenic, added hormones, and antibiotics; worsening soil quality; and an increasing lack of biodiversity. Supporters of organics say that if these elements were factored into conventional food prices, consumers would pay less in comparison for organics.

Another reason organic food is more expensive, advocates say, is that the U.S. government pays subsidies to conventional growers. The money keeps prices low in the grocery stores even though consumers eventually pay for the subsidies through increased taxes. According to supporters of organics foods, this amounts to corporate welfare for big agribusiness from the USDA and the federal government.

Over time, the formula for subsidies based on crop type and volume have changed; now two commodities, corn and soybeans, receive over 70 percent of the earmarked federal funds. USDA statistics for the period from 1995 to 2003 showed that three-quarters of the subsidies went to the top 10 percent of growers. In other words, the government subsidies supported big industrial operations rather than small family farms.[10] In 2007, Indiana Senator Richard Lugar criticized those subsidies, still in place today, and said they hurt the family farmer. The Federal Farm bill that governs subsidies was originally introduced after the Great Depression as a way to alleviate poverty among small farmers and rural communities.

HEALTH

Americans who choose organic foods say the reason is simple: they want food that is better for them. Supporters of organics are concerned about eating conventionally grown crops with pesticide residues, dairy with growth hormones, and livestock fed with antibiotics. FDA figures show that half of the produce currently tested in grocery stores contains measurable residues of pesticides. Even more alarming, laboratory test results from the FDA Pesticide Residue Monitoring Program showed that eight popular baby foods brands tested positive for the presence of 16 pesticides, including three carcinogens.[11]

Of the 900 or so active ingredients in pesticides legally allowed in the United States, some 20 have been shown to cause cancer in animals and are classified as possible human carcinogens. Unfortunately, there are no studies to measure the risk to American consumers from eating pesticide residues. According to Aaron Blair, an epidemiologist at the National Cancer Institute (NCI), "I don't know any epidemiologic studies that tell you what the risk from pesticides in food is for an adult."[12]

However, scientists are looking closely at the effects of pesticides on infants and children. In May 2007, many of the world's leading environmental scientists met to highlight their research at a conference led by Philippe Grandjean of the Department of Environmental Medicine of the Institute of Public Health at the University of Southern Denmark. Based on their findings, the scientists warned that babies exposed to chemicals including pesticides may be more susceptible to attention deficit disorder, asthma, and cancer, and that this early exposure may lead to increased susceptibility to diseases later in life.[13]

Various government agencies have also taken note of potential problems for children from pesticide exposure. The Environmental Protection Agency (EPA) and the National Academy of Sciences cautioned parents that standard chemical pesticides are up to 10 times more toxic to children than to adults, depending on body weight. The developing organ systems of young children are highly vulnerable and less able to detoxify chemicals than adult systems. A government study released in 2003 looked at blood samples of children aged two to four, and found that concentrations of pesticide residues were six times higher in children eating conventionally farmed fruits and vegetables compared with those eating organic food.[14]

Supporters of organic foods suspect that evidence of the long-term effects of pesticides is now being seen in children of all ages. According to the U.S. Department of Health and Human Services (HHS), organophosphate pesticides are found in the blood of 95 percent of Americans tested. Those organophosphate pesticide levels are also twice as high in blood samples from children as from adults. According to HHS, exposure to pesticides is linked to hyperactivity, behavior disorders, learning disabilities, developmental delays, and motor dysfunction. HHS noted that organophosphate pesticide chemicals account for half of the insecticides used in the United States.[15]

Pesticides were developed to kill insects that harm crops. Unfortunately, those pests are never completely eliminated, because spraying density varies within a field; bugs get different doses at the edge of the field versus the middle of the field, and so forth. Some insects get a lethal dose and die; others have a natural resistance to the chemicals and live. If that resistance is genetic, it is passed on and becomes more prevalent in the next generation. Eventually, the insect population consists only of immune insects. More than 500 species of insects now resist chemicals, and some 300 weed species resist all herbicides, making a large number of pesticides and herbicides ineffective.

Does it work to just spray more? Historical usage patterns and their effects on crop losses illustrate that more spraying does not translate into improved or more abundant crops. In 1948, farmers used 50 million pounds of pesticides and measured about a 7 percent loss of field crops. In 2000, growers sprayed nearly one billion pounds of pesticides, yet crop losses were almost double at 13 percent.[16] The bottom line is that organically grown produce is safer than conventional produce when it comes to pesticide residues, and U.S. consumers who want to avoid pesticides are choosing organic foods in growing numbers.

NUTRITIONAL VALUES

Are organic fruits and vegetables more nutritious than their conventional counterparts? According to a state of science analysis released in 2008 by the Organic Center, organic foods provide a clear advantage in macronutrients and in micronutrients. Researchers led by Charles Benbrook, former executive director of the Board of Agriculture of the National Academy of Sciences, concluded that "the average serving of organic plant-based food contains about 25 percent more of the nutrients encompassed in the study than a comparable-sized serving of the same food produced by conventional farming methods."[17] Although the two-year project focused on plant foods, it also suggested that there was strong evidence that poultry and livestock raised on organic food produced meat, milk, and eggs with higher levels of protein, more vitamins and minerals, and improved levels of heart-healthy fats.

Studies indicate that although grass-fed beef is as high in saturated fat as conventional beef, it also has higher levels of good fats, the omega-3 fatty acids that come from the grass. The meat from organic cattle also contains more vitamin E and other vitamins from the nutrients in the grass. The animals eat the low-calorie grass and move around, unlike cattle jammed into feedlots eating corn and feed mixed with antibiotics and hormones. Grass-fed cattle also have lower levels of bacteria such as *E. coli* and *Campylobacter* than feedlot animals. As a final benefit, grass-fed cattle do not have to digest the concentrated fats, proteins, and carbohydrates in corn and soybeans; they get sick less frequently and receive fewer antibiotic treatments, resulting in less antibiotic residue in their meat.

Research also found that organic milk contains more vitamins, essential fats, and antioxidants than conventionally produced milk. A Danish research team published their findings in 2005 at a conference in England, and announced that their three-year project, funded by the European Union, found unexpectedly high levels of nutrients in organic milk as compared with conventional milk—50 percent higher in vitamin E, 75 percent higher in betacarotene, and two to three times higher in antioxidants.[18] On the other hand, drinking conventionally produced and processed milk may have serious health effects, especially for young children. Following tests on 788 samples of milk by the USDA in 2005, the agency reported residues of an average of 2.5 pesticides per sample. There were also residues of synthetic insecticides and other toxins in nearly half of the samples of conventional milk.[19]

All vegetables are not created equal; how a plant is grown, the soil it grows in, and what is added or taken away from the soil all play a part in the quality of the food being grown. Supporters of organic farming suggest that the heavy use of artificial fertilizers is a self-perpetuating cycle: the more used, the more sterile the soil becomes, and the greater the amount of fertilizer needed to achieve the same crop results. This pattern finally reaches a plateau, where production levels off or starts to fall despite larger and larger applications of fertilizer.

Scientists are also looking at other problems associated with chemical fertilizers. For example, adding phosphorus may kill tiny filaments of fungi that assist plants in absorbing nutrients from the soil. The NPK fertilizer used by conventional farmers (the P is phosphorus) helps plants grow, but diminishes other soil qualities including these fungi, which may ultimately deplete the nutritional value of the fruit or vegetable.

Organic farming reduces pollutants in the groundwater and adds to rather than subtracts from the soil, according to the Organic Trade Association. Organic farming decreases pesticide use and uses less energy than conventional farming. Supporters of organic farming say that the main advantages of artificial fertilizers over natural sources are that they come in a bag, are easier to apply, and have a guaranteed and measured composition. However, when weighed against the effects they ultimately have on soil, robbing it of its fertility, those advantages pale in comparison.

Conversely, critics of organics suggest that organic vegetables, meat, and eggs are more likely to be contaminated with *E. coli* or other bacteria than conventional products. Organic farmers use manure as fertilizer, which critics say is a possible source of contamination. Experts caution that there is always the possibility of contamination from many sources, especially human hands, no matter how clean a farm may be. Fruits or vegetables that are cut up and handled are an even more likely source.

Organic farmers in most cases use compost that includes manure aged and heat-treated in a process based on strict guidelines set up by the USDA. Any raw manure applied to fields must be put down at least 120 days before harvest so bacteria will die out long before the crop is gathered. Conventional farms do not have to follow this rule, and can apply raw manure much closer to harvest time.

Still, critics of organics point to the three people who died, and the hundreds sickened in over 26 states, by *E. coli*–tainted spinach in the fall of 2007 as an example of the dangers of organic produce. When officials determined the point of origin and the specific product carrying the *E. coli*, they discovered that the culprit was triple-washed, bagged fresh spinach grown on land leased by an organic food company and packaged by a leader in the organic industry, Selections Foods (whose organic brands include Earthbound Farms). Although the land was in a transitional stage, in the process of becoming a certified organic farm, investigators were not able to determine how the *E. coli* got into the spinach. They did find the same strain of bacteria in river water and in cattle and pigs on a ranch within a mile of the fields where the spinach was grown.

FEASIBILITY

A key objection to organic farming comes from opponents who maintain that it is not economically or technologically feasible to feed the world's growing population using organic fertilizers or chemical-free pest control. To address world hunger, they argue, nations such as the United States must produce tons of food, and the only way to do that efficiently is by employing highly mechanized technology and chemical pesticides and herbicides. Yet studies that compare organic and chemical-intensive systems show increasing organic yields. Researchers at the University of Wisconsin released the results of a 12-year study in the March–April 2008 issue of *Agronomy Journal;* they found that organic systems were as productive as conventional systems when it came to producing alfalfa and wheat, and were as effective most of the time for corn and soybeans.[20]

Earlier, the results of a 21-year Swiss study released and published in the May 31, 2002 issue of *Science* showed that even though organic crop yields had been from 10 to 20 percent lower than conventional yields, they only required one half as much energy and fertilizer as conventional crops, and needed 97 percent fewer pesticides. The organic soils also retained greater fertility and biological activity, which had a positive effect all the way up the food chain to birds and larger animals.[21]

ORGANIC FAST FOOD

Whether Americans believe or reject the possible benefits of organics, it's obvious they are here to stay. In fact, besides their explosive growth in major supermarkets, organics are now showing up in fast-food restaurants. Is organic fast food an oxymoron? Not according to Gary Hirshberg, who says it's possible to provide tasty, natural fast food. Hirshberg, who founded Stonyfield Yogurt, came up with the idea for his O'Naturals fast-food restaurant after he and his family struggled to find something to eat at fast food restaurants during various outings. With six locations in places as far-flung as Portland, Maine and Orlando, Florida, the New England–based chain offers organics in at least one-third of its menu items. O'Naturals choices include sandwiches made with wild Alaskan salmon, free range and grass-fed organic beef, and free-roaming chickens.

Organic fast food is priced higher than conventional fast food, but supporters say it is a clear example of paying for quality over quantity. For example, the O'Naturals Wrangler sandwich, made with organic roast beef, Swiss cheese, rosemary, onions, organic lettuce, and tomato on flatbread, comes at twice the price of a Big Mac. But Hirshberg is betting Americans are willing to pay for convenient food that is clearly healthier than a Big Mac or a Whopper and fries. Along with sandwiches, other O'Naturals menu items include stir-fry noodles, a host of soups such as carrot ginger or white bean and escarole, and smoothies, organic milk, coffee, and tea.

Supporters of organics credit the Whole Foods grocery store chain as an early leader in successful, organic fast food. The store, which opened in Texas in 1980, became the first national certified organic grocer in the United States in 2003, and posted sales that year of over three billion dollars. The prepared food section in any of the 270 stores is filled daily with businesspeople grabbing lunch from a salad bar piled high with fresh, organic vegetables and toppings or sandwiches from a deli section where items are packaged to go or prepared while customers wait. For those who have the time, tables are even available for sit-down eating. After Whole Foods got the ball rolling, others, including O'Naturals, have followed close behind.

Organic to Go, a Seattle based company founded in 2004, recently picked up four local cafés and a small catering operation from the Washington DC–based High Noon restaurants. This gives Organic to Go locations on the West Coast in Seattle, Los Angeles, and San Diego, plus three café locations in the District of Columbia and one in Virginia, for a total of 33 cafes. High Noon owner Mark Ordan sold his Fresh Fields grocery chain of 22 stores to Whole Foods in 1996, and opened High Noon in the busy downtown DC business area. With the purchase of the Washington locations, Organic to Go now calls itself "America's first fast-casual café certified organic retailer," and offers organic food whenever possible. According to the company's Web site, at a minimum its products are made with natural ingredients free from harmful additives, and made with organic ingredients whenever possible.

Others are also bringing organic fast food to the DC area. Three Georgetown University graduates opened a restaurant called Sweetgreen in the Georgetown section of the city in 2007. Customers choose organic greens, arugula, or mesclun mix, along with veggie toppings and crunchy options such as croutons or candied nuts. The to-go packaging for each salad is biodegradable.

How to Avoid Pesticides

American consumers who want to buy organic products and reduce their pesticide exposure can now find plenty of choices to meet their needs and their budgets. Keep in mind that the more a food is processed, the less health value its organic version may offer, as with cereals, pastas, or other processed foods. Some produce is likely to have higher pesticide residue levels when eaten fresh if the skin is consumed as well. The banana is an example of a fruit that, when peeled, loses any pesticide residue.

The Environmental Working Group (EWG), a nonprofit consumer activist group, looked at government statistics on pesticide residues for a number of fruits and vegetables. They strongly recommend that consumers reduce their pesticide exposure and avoid their "Dirty Dozen," the twelve most contaminated fruits and vegetables, even if they don't buy organics. Among fruits, nectarines had the highest percentage testing positive for pesticide residue, whereas peaches and red raspberries had the most pesticides on a single sample. For vegetables, celery and spinach carried the most pesticides, and spinach had the most residue on a single sample. The dozen also include apples, sweet bell peppers, strawberries, cherries, pears, imported grapes, lettuce and potatoes. On the flip side, those twelve fruits and vegetables with the least contamination are onions, avocados, frozen sweet corn, pineapples, mangoes, asparagus, frozen sweet peas, kiwifruit, bananas, cabbage, broccoli, and papaya.

THE FUTURE OF ORGANICS

Americans are willing to pay for something they place a high value on, but they are extremely value conscious consumers. What does that mean for organic food? Stores such as Whole Foods and Trader Joe's are thriving, thanks in part to their ability to sell at increasing volumes, while offering organic products at lower prices. Consumers who buy organic food are saying they do not want to be part of an ongoing science experiment. There is little government research aimed at identifying any long-term effects of eating pesticide residues, even though these resides are found in measurable levels on fruits and vegetables and in the bloodstream. Supporters of organics say they are willing to pay more to avoid this unknown. Given the number of pesticides banned over the years for health and environmental reasons, this appears to be a reasonable choice, especially concerning young children.

Buying and eating organic food has also come to be seen as a personal statement, a show of support for the environment. Organic farming is a way to push back at industrialized agriculture with its huge monocrops, massive energy consumption, and overindulgence in pesticides. Unfortunately, as the demand for organic food grows, that growth actually threatens organic ideals, and has led to the split between little and big organics. At risk are the small organic growers, victims of a capitalist system that demands they grow big or be bought up by corporations such as Wal-Mart or Costco.

Ironically, the appeal of organic ideals, small farms, and sustainable agriculture sparked the popularity that could now put small organic producers out of business. Up to 57 percent of organic shoppers now buy their food at mainstream grocery stores and discounters rather than smaller health food stores, according to statistics from the Food Marketing Institute.[22] Supporters of organics hope the growing number of Americans attracted to organic food will eventually strengthen the movement rather than compromise its standards, and provide enough buyers to keep everyone in business.

At the same time, other consumers are opting out of the mainstream food industry and turning to more direct sources for organic food. Rising numbers of Americans interested in supporting small organic farms now buy directly from farmers or local farmers' markets. These community-supported agriculture programs (CSAs) are literally growing like weeds across the country. For a yearly or monthly fee, members receive fresh, organic produce throughout the growing season. Some CSAs allow members to work; others just have customers pick up their weekly order. For example, one week's order might include broccoli, peppers, zucchini, and melon but not out-of-season produce such as potatoes, grapes, or strawberries.

This emerging alternative food economy is jointly driven by farmers taking control of their shrinking markets, and consumers focused on getting fresh, healthy, organic food that does not have to be shipped thousands of miles. In fact, the rising popularity of organic food and this movement to support sustainable, local agriculture has sometimes resulted in the demand for local, organic produce outstripping supply. Will the power of this alternative food economy be able to shape Americans' opinions about the benefits of organic food? Although no one can be absolutely certain of the outcome, supporters of organics hope time will prove them right before too much damage is done to the environment—and our food supply.

CHAPTER 9

From the Field to the Table: How Safe Is Our Food?

The term "food safety" is a relative one, and in twenty-first-century America, it is no longer just about potato salad left out in the sun or hamburgers not cooked enough on the grill. Today, American consumers must contend with nationwide outbreaks of foodborne illness and tainted foods from countries such as China and Mexico, and at the same time weigh the effects of pesticides, poisonous metals, growth hormones, genetically modified foods, and irradiation.

Unlike our European counterparts, until recent years Americans had shown only modest concerns about foodborne illness, and even less interest in related safety issues such as pesticides or the overuse of antibiotics in livestock feed. However, that laid-back attitude is changing, according to a recent national survey that showed that three-quarters of Americans polled were more concerned about the food they eat today than they were five years ago, and 57 percent said they had stopped eating certain foods following a food scare.[1]

As the U.S. food industry works overtime to influence what and how much people eat to preserve the economic health of their industry, Americans struggle to practice healthy nutrition by eating more fresh fruits and vegetables. Unfortunately, industry profits and food safety don't always work well together. Consumers have every right to be worried about the safety of their food. Statistics from the Centers for Disease Control and Prevention (CDC) show that some 76 million Americans are stricken with foodborne diseases each year.

The CDC serves as the lead federal agency for conducting disease surveillance and outbreak investigation. It estimates that, of those millions of foodborne disease cases each year, approximately 325,000 Americans require hospitalization, and 5,000 die.[2] Sadly, many other victims, of all ages, races, and economic levels, suffer bouts of vomiting and diarrhea never realizing they have a foodborne illness. The CDC estimates that 20 illnesses caused by *E. coli* O157:H7 and 38 cases of salmonellosis occur for every case that is officially reported to federal public health authorities.[3]

Politicians and government officials call our country's food supply one of the safest in the world. Yet if that is the case, why are so many Americans getting sick from peanut butter, beef, raw spinach, strawberries, cantaloupe, ice cream, fruit juice, peppers, and many other foods? The summer of 2008 will be remembered for an outbreak of *Salmonella* that sickened at least 1,440 people across the United States and was called the worst foodborne outbreak in at least a decade. Although the early evidence suggested that the bacteria traced to fresh tomatoes from Florida, the CDC and Food and Drug Administration (FDA) ultimately placed the blame on serrano and jalapeño peppers grown in Mexico.

The outbreak began in late April; most cases appeared during May and June. Texas accounted for nearly 40 percent of all confirmed cases, a fact that eventually persuaded investigators to shift focus from the Florida-grown tomatoes to the Mexican peppers. The fact that illnesses occurred in multiple states also suggested that contamination had likely occurred early in the distribution chain. The joint investigation by the CDC and FDA eventually found strong evidence that the jalapeño peppers were a major carrier of this particular strain of *Salmonella*, and that serrano peppers were a secondary carrier; both came from farms that sent produce to a common packing facility in Mexico. From there, the peppers were shipped to the United States.

A *Salmonella* outbreak of that size is not cheap. The Economic Research Service (ERS) of the U.S. Department of Agriculture (USDA) estimates that the economic cost of salmonellosis alone in 2007 was over $2 billion dollars. In calculating this figure, the ERS measured medical expenses, lost work, and premature death.[4] The figure did not include associated costs, such as care for extended medical complications or pain and suffering. In other words, foodborne illnesses significantly costs the United States every year in both lives and dollars.

Salmonella is one culprit; however, it is far from the only food safety issue. The United States imports about 40 percent of its fresh produce, a figure that continues to go up. This globalization of the nation's food supply means the average American eats about 260 pounds of imported foods each year.[5] Even though many of the outbreaks of foodborne illness come from meat, vegetables, and fruit produced in the United States, China's melamine scandal raised serious doubts about the safety of imports.

In 2008, dairy products from China were recalled around the world after they were found to contain melamine, a dangerous industrial chemical that artificially inflates protein content when added to a food. In China, the melamine-tainted milk killed four babies and sickened 54,000 children. Later that year, Wal-Mart pulled a brand of eggs from all its stores in China after tests discovered they were tainted with the same toxic chemical blamed for sickening the babies. The discovery of melamine in eggs raised a serious question about how deeply the chemical had penetrated China's food chain.

The reality for Americans is that food can be contaminated anywhere from the field to the table. Given the miles and processing it now passes through, consumers need to ask important questions about foreign producers. Do they use pesticides or additives banned in the United States, or have more relaxed food handling and inspection rules than this country? These invisible pesticides and other toxins are as serious a hazard as the foodborne pathogens, bacteria, viruses, and parasites in restaurants and home kitchens.

With more U.S. meals being consumed away from home at fast-food and sit-down restaurants, Americans want a food supply that is as safe as possible. To define what that means, this chapter will explore the most pressing U.S. food safety issues and look at the history of foodborne illness. It will detail government regulations and proposed changes in those laws, and consider future legislation. Finally, because food is produced, processed, shipped, sold, and often cooked before it is eaten, the chapter will introduce consumer groups who work to keep food industry lobbyists in check, and will include updated food safety suggestions and practices.

The outbreak of food poisoning from peppers in the summer of 2008 was not an isolated incident. In 1992, the fast food restaurant Jack in the Box was another canary in the coalmine, forcing federal agencies to recognize the need for improvements in commercial food safety regulations. In the case of Jack in the Box, 732 people became ill and four children died due to deadly *E. coli* 0157:H7 in the meat. Public health officials eventually traced the contaminated beef patties back to their supplier, but not before hundreds of people were hospitalized and dozens of children suffered kidney failure. Their kidneys stopped working due to a serious urinary tract infection, known as hemolyric uremic syndrome, caused by *E. coli*.

Jack in the Box officials responded by recalling all the meat and offering to pay all hospital costs for consumers sickened by their burgers. They also discovered that the hamburger had not been cooked enough to kill the *E. coli*. An investigation by the Washington State Health Department showed that the burgers may have been heated to between 120 degrees and

140 degrees, a figure well below the required the 155 degrees. Although cooking the meat thoroughly might have prevented the Jack in the Box tragedy, consumer advocates called it a clear warning; the time had come to revamp the 90-year-old food safety regulations, and especially how the government inspected meat. It was also apparent that food safety was not just the responsibility of home cooks or the USDA. Consumer groups challenged food producers, processors, and sellers to stop expecting the government to shoulder the entire burden of national food safety, and to shift their focus from improving profit margins to improving safety.

HISTORY OF REGULATIONS

As early as the 1860s, the safety of the nation's meat supply was a growing public health concern. In response to the problem, President Abraham Lincoln signed legislation in 1862 to create the U.S. Department of Agriculture. Later, as the country continued its westward expansion, President Chester Arthur recognized the need to work with ranchers and meatpackers to eradicate livestock diseases. He signed the Bureau of Animal Industry Act in 1884, which created the USDA's Bureau of Animal Industry, the forerunner of the Food Safety and Inspection Service (FSIS). Today, the FSIS has a leading role in the nation's food safety system.

By the end of the nineteenth century, the nation's slaughterhouses were the target of muckraking journalists whose stories of filth and disease terrified American consumers as well as our European trade partners. To quiet criticism of the nation's meat handling practices, Congress passed the Meat Inspection Act in 1890. That legislation authorized inspection of salt pork, bacon, and pigs for export. However, the law, and others that followed, did not calm overseas worries about the safety of U.S. meat exports. This unease about the quality of American meat has been a recurrent theme in U.S. exports for decades. For example, in the summer of 2008, thousands of South Koreans rioted in the streets of Seoul to stop the import of American beef into their country.

Things went from bad to worse in 1905, when the government faced an avalanche of U.S. consumer protests following the publication of Upton Sinclair's novel, *The Jungle*. In his book, Sinclair awakened the nation to real dangers in the food supply. He wrote in excruciating detail about the filthy conditions in Chicago meatpacking plants. The story focused on an immigrant who at one point described how, after the government inspectors left for the day, the "downers"—the sick, diseased, and injured cattle—were butchered: "It took a couple of hours to get them out of the way, and in the end Jurgis saw them go into the chilling rooms with the rest of the meat, being carefully scattered here and there so that they could not be identified."[6]

The book, combined with the efforts of the FDA and its director, Dr. Harvey Washington Wiley, pushed food safety to center stage. Wiley made national headlines in 1902 when he recruited young men to act as guinea pigs and test different food additives. The "poison squad" ate meals made with ingredients such as borax, salicylic acid, formaldehyde, sulphuric acid, sodium benzoate, and copper salts. Drawn into the debates over food safety, President Theodore Roosevelt and the Congress brought the 1906 Pure Food and Drug Act and the Federal Meat Inspection Act (FMIA) into law.

The FMIA called for the USDA to inspect meat largely by looking, touching, or poking and smelling the meat. The law was designed by Congress to prevent sick animals from getting into American food; no one imagined a time when they would need to check for microscopic pathogens. The act also called for the USDA to appoint government inspectors, with some trained as veterinarians, to work in every U.S. slaughterhouse in operation at that time. However, the law kept inspectors from looking at the entire livestock operation from field to table. Instead, the government could only examine the animals in the slaughterhouse; they were not allowed to check livestock at any other point. The law also left the USDA with no ability to recall tainted food once it left the plant. Those omissions continue to frustrate consumer advocates as well as government agencies, because under the current laws, the USDA and FDA continue to lack the specific recall authority available to other government agencies responsible for the safety of products such as toys, heart pacemakers, and automobiles. Those agencies may order a recall and impose monetary penalties if a company violates recall requirements, but neither the USDA nor FDA can order a company to recall potentially unsafe food. They also cannot fine a company that is slow to conduct a food recall or provides inaccurate customer lists.

The FMIA set up basic sanitary rules for the meatpacking industry: mandatory inspection of livestock before slaughter, mandatory inspection of every carcass after death, and explicit sanitary standards for each slaughterhouse. In 1906, the USDA hired more than 1,300 inspectors to carry out the inspections at some 163 slaughterhouses across the nation; by 1907, the government employed more than 2,200 inspectors at approximately 700 establishments.[7] At the same time, "Typhoid Mary" Mallon, an Irish immigrant cook, introduced Americans to a different aspect of foodborne illness. She was a carrier of the typhoid bacteria, but did not get sick. Instead, she passed the disease on and sickened many of her employers and their families. At the time, she was called the most dangerous woman in America, and was quarantined on Ellis Island. Her confinement, along with the 1906 acts, continued to keep food safety in the news.

Surprisingly, the 1906 FMIA did not address chicken slaughterhouses, because at the time Americans were buying what few chickens they ate directly from farms. Consumer demand for poultry did not increase until after World War II. One factor that kept U.S. chicken consumption low was a 1920 outbreak of avian influenza in New York City, which had been the hub of poultry distribution for the United States. By 1957, when the demand for chicken picked up, the USDA recommended that poultry processing plants only buy chickens from producers who voluntarily met USDA sanitation requirements. It wasn't long before Congress passed the Poultry Products Inspection Act (PPIA) of 1957. The new inspection requirements for poultry mirrored those for cattle and pigs—rules such as sanitary standards for processing facilities, and before-and-after inspections. Once again, inspection methods included using sight, touch, and smell, but paid no attention to microscopic bacteria.

Decades earlier, typhoid fever, cholera, botulism, and trichinosis were common. However, they had disappeared in the United States thanks to pasteurization, improved canning, and food preservation techniques. On the other hand, increasingly large livestock production practices created new problems. The Food Safety and Inspection Service (FSIS) was established in 1981 to monitor the handling of all U.S. meat, poultry, and egg products as critics began to call for tougher inspection methods that tested for invisible pathogens. Eggs were a perfect example: by the 1980s, disease-causing microbes had developed inside chickens and passed into the eggs.

The connection between *Salmonella* and poultry intensified, and in the 1990s U.S. scientists publicly acknowledged that laying hens were carrying *Salmonella enteritidis* internally. The increase in contaminated eggs was linked to U.S. industrial farming practices and to the crowded conditions of laying hens. With so many birds in such close quarters, the bacteria were easily passed from one hen to another. Many chickens had infected ovaries even though they showed no signs of sickness, and the infected birds shed the bacteria into the egg white. Once the shell was secreted around the egg white, the bacteria was invisibly sealed inside the egg. This situation was extremely rare in the 1960s and 1970s, but by the 1990s the number of cases of *Salmonella enteritidis* infection from transovarian transfer had increased dramatically.

The situation exploded in 1994 when more than 200,000 people got food poisoning from contaminated ice cream.[8] It was a massive job for the government to track down the common factor among hundreds of thousands of people, but officials finally pinpointed a specific brand of ice cream as the cause. The product was recalled. Researchers discovered that the ice cream had been transported by tanker trucks that previously carried unpasteurized eggs. Those eggs were infected with *Salmonella*. Today, the USDA estimates that more than 70 billion eggs are sold each year in U.S. stores, and that 19 percent contain *Salmonella* bacteria.[9] This means that American consumers are buying millions of *Salmonella*-infected eggs each year. In 2006, the FSIS implemented a "*Salmonella* attack plan" to try to lower the rate of infection in U.S. eggs.

A FEDERAL MAZE

A look at current federal food safety responsibilities reveals a mishmash of agencies and laws. There are as many as 12 government agencies with at least a small regulatory role in the foods Americans eat. However, the two main agencies responsible for the safety of our food are the U.S. Department of Agriculture (USDA) and the U.S. Food and Drug Administration (FDA). The USDA, through the FSIS, regulates meat, poultry and processed egg products along with foods that contain them. It also oversees pasteurized egg products.

The FDA, which works on food safety chiefly through its Center for Food Safety and Applied Nutrition (CFSAN), has the lead responsibility for administering food safety regulations. The agency addresses the safety of all other foods, including fresh fruits and vegetables, milk, eggs, and any processed foods that do not contain meat, poultry, or processed egg products. It also oversees canned and imported foods, some 80 percent of the nation's food supply. This creates a complicated system of checks and balances. For example, the USDA regulates spaghetti sauce with meat stock, but the FDA regulates spaghetti sauce without meat stock. The USDA oversees pizza with meat toppings; the FDA inspects the safety of cheese pizza. The USDA performs daily slaughterhouse inspections, whereas the FDA only inspects plants in its jurisdiction once every five years.

Eggs and egg products are a prime example of complex government regulations at work. Basically, the FDA is responsible for inspecting shell eggs but not hen houses. The USDA divides responsibilities for eggs between the Animal and Plant Health Inspection Service (APHIS), which oversees animal health; the Agricultural Marketing Service, which grades eggs for size and quality but does not check their safety; and the Food Safety and Inspection Service (FSIS), which inspects liquid, frozen, and powdered egg products but not shell eggs. With no single agency assigned to monitor overall egg safety, frequent infections occur and consumers end up suffering the consequences.

At the same time, in recent years, the FDA office in charge of food safety has had its workload increased, its budget cut, and its number of employees reduced. According to the Government Accountability Office, the FDA's Center for Food Safety and Applied Nutrition saw its budget drop 14 percent from 2003 to 2006.[10] The FDA is now conducting half the food-safety inspections it did 10 years ago, with fewer and fewer inspectors in the field. The number of food-import inspectors has also dropped about 20 percent, while food imports have climbed. Figures show that just over one percent of fish, vegetables, fruit, and other imported foods were inspected by the FDA in the spring of 2007.[11] This spells trouble for American consumers: as problems with melamine in Chinese dairy products and *Salmonella* in Mexican peppers illustrated, imports are a growing food safety concern for the nation.

In recent years, FDA inspections discovered a number of problems with other products from China, including frozen catfish tainted with veterinary drugs, fresh ginger polluted with pesticides, and melons contaminated with toxins. Federal records also suggest that China is not the only country with food export problems. In 2007, government inspectors seized more food shipments from India and Mexico than from China, according to the *New York Times*.[12] To deal more effectively with the growing volume of imports, the FDA and the USDA have adopted an inspection philosophy that prioritizes foods, sources, or producers they suspect represent the biggest risk to public health. Basically, these agencies only have the resources to examine a fraction of the food products imported into the United States.

CHANGES IN REGULATIONS

Beginning in October 2008, a new federal rule took effect requiring retailers to identify the country of origin when labeling imported foods. Consumers worried about lax safety regulations can avoid imports from any country they want—sort of. The country-of-origin labeling (COOL) law designates where items originated, from Chile to the United States. However, labels aren't required for processed foods or mixed foods. This means that cantaloupe slices from Guatemala or Mexico would have labels, but a frozen pea and carrot mix would not. Plain raw chicken would be labeled, but not breaded chicken tenders. Bagged lettuce could be labeled, but if radicchio was added, no label is required.

The COOL law passed in 2002, but large meatpackers and other food industry lobbyists persuaded Congress to delay implementation. In 2005, seafood labeling was phased in, but the 2008 law exempts meat and seafood sold in butcher shops and fish markets. There is also a conflict between large meat producers and smaller operations that only process American raised livestock. The large operations argue that it's too expensive to separate cattle from various countries. At least one major corporation, Tyson Fresh Meats, suggested labeling their beef "Product of the U.S., Canada or Mexico." The National Farmers Union is protesting and the USDA is considering the situation.

Jean Halloran of Consumers Union has said that the COOL law is "a very good thing because we'll have a lot more information," but she cautioned that consumers can still be fooled given all the exceptions.[13] She suggested that the labels will help consumers worried about safety regulations in certain countries to avoid imported food from those areas. Another benefit is the additional information readily available for people who suspect they have food poisoning; they could potentially help investigators pinpoint the origin of suspicious foods thanks to the new labels. Stores that violate the law can be fined.

The COOL law is one of several food safety changes inspired by poisoning tragedies involving imported foods. On the domestic front, the government agreed with consumer advocates and put a new system using research and technology into place following the Jack in the Box outbreak of *E. coli*. Designed to be more than a scientific version of the "poke and sniff" method already used by inspectors, the Hazard Analysis and Critical Control Point (HACCP) program puts the responsibility for safety on food processors and producers, requiring them to identify points in their production line where there is an increased risk of contamination. The HACCP system also requires the use of steam and acid carcass washes to protect against invisible pathogens. Although the fundamental principles of the HACCP program offer a sound tool for companies to improve food safety, consumer advocates say that, in practice, the program is often used as a substitute for government inspection, rather than the two systems working in tandem.

The HACCP concept was developed in the 1960s when the U.S. National Aeronautics and Space Administration (NASA) needed safe food for space flights. Today, meat and poultry HACCP systems are regulated by the USDA, and seafood and juice HACCP systems are regulated by the FDA. The seafood rules were finalized in 1995, the final rule for the juice industry took effect in 2002, and the USDA rules for meat and poultry processing were finalized in 1999. To help sort out which regulations would be feasible, the FSIS first conducted a pilot program with volunteer food companies. Data collected from the project showed significant improvements in both food safety and other consumer protections, according to the FSIS.

There are two overall types of procedures in the HACCP program: carcass inspection and verification inspection. Government and industry experts agree that identifying and preventing hazards that could cause foodborne illness has improved overall food safety. Carcass inspection requires inspectors, stationed on the slaughter line at a fixed location, to view the meat postmortem. Meanwhile, the verification inspector examines plant records as well as microbial samples of the meat for testing and analysis. Since the HACCP system has been initiated in the United States, the severity of food poisoning incidents remains a problem, but the overall number of cases of listeriosis and salmonellosis is on the decline.

However, beginning in 2007, scientists noted an increase in the prevalence of *E. coli* in beef products. By mid-October of 2008, USDA meat inspectors had recorded a 50 percent increase in contaminated beef samples over the number from the same time in the previous year.[14] Although their findings are not conclusive, researchers are testing whether the use of an ethanol product called distillers grain in cattle feed may be connected with the increase in contaminated beef. Scientists say there is still a lot they do not understand about the bacteria, and federal efforts to improve slaughterhouse safety will continue.

Additional Food Safety Issues

The FDA instituted a Produce Safety Action Plan in 2004 that built on the HACCP program. As part of the plan, the FDA provided technical assistance to the food industry in addressing microbial hazards for five food groups: cantaloupes, lettuce and leafy greens, tomatoes, green onions, and fresh herbs. Other actions taken by the FDA to improve food safety include a legally binding safety limit for polychlorinated biphenyls (PCBs), and guidelines for safety limits for six pesticides as well as for mercury, paralytic shellfish poison, and histamine in canned tuna. Histamine is the chemical responsible for scombroid poisoning, a common type of seafood poisoning often misdiagnosed because it resembles an allergic reaction.

One area consumer advocates want more government oversight in is the use of antibiotics in livestock feed, which in turn could improve the nation's growing problem of antibiotic resistance. Antibiotics were first given to livestock to accelerate growth, but as more and more animals were crowded into smaller areas, the antibiotics were also used to hold at bay diseases that would cut into producer's profits. A sick cow cannot legally be slaughtered in a U.S. slaughter house. Some estimates show that the volume of antibiotics used in animal feed equals or exceeds that used in human medicine.

U.S. livestock feed holds another potentially fatal food safety hazard. In April 2008, the FDA issued a final regulation to keep certain cattle parts from all animal feed in an effort to protect American consumers from bovine spongiform encephalopathy (BSE), also known as mad cow disease. BSE spread in Great Britain in the 1990s when cattle were fed bone meal and meat from other animals that had the disease.

The new FDA measure restricts the addition of cattle brains and spinal cords to U.S. animal feed if the parts are from cattle older than 30 months of age. Carcasses of cattle not inspected by the FDA are also prohibited from being ground up and put into cattle feed if the animals are older than 30 months of age. The FDA maintains that the risk of BSE in cattle less than 30 months of age is low, and that their parts can be used in feed with minimal risk of infection. The United States is one of the few countries in the world that allows any animal parts in livestock feed, a fact that for years prompted South Korea to ban imports of U.S. beef. The South Korean government only recently decided to allow American beef after U.S. government officials increased funding for several aspects of BSE control. Specifically, the USDA, through the Food Safety and Inspection Service (FSIS), received an extra four million dollars in the 2005 federal budget to improve how it monitored BSE regulations, and the Agricultural Research Service was awarded another five million dollars to develop better BSE-testing technologies.[15]

TECHNOLOGICAL INNOVATIONS

Irradiation of food to kill pathogens, genetically modified crops whose genes are altered to improve resistance to insects and pesticides, and growth hormones used to increase milk production in dairy cows are technological innovations considered important food safety issues by American consumer advocates. Whether these and other developments represent a danger depends on viewpoint. In general, government agencies and scientists support these technologies as tools to promote food safety and combat world hunger, whereas critics oppose them as untested and potentially dangerous.

Irradiation

Ironically, irradiation of food began as a way to use nuclear technology to solve the problems caused by that technology itself. The idea originated in 1953, when President Dwight Eisenhower gave his "Atoms for Peace" address to encourage the world to use atomic energy and its waste products in positive ways. However, right from the start, American consumers were skeptical of the idea of treating food with radiation, especially following World War II and the use of the atomic bomb. Nonetheless, the government kept moving the program forward, and in 1963 the FDA approved irradiation to kill insects in wheat and flour. The FDA then approved irradiation to kill growth sprouts in potatoes in 1964.

Controversy arose in 1968, when the FDA rejected a petition to use radiation to sterilize canned bacon, reporting noticeable problems in animal studies that raised doubts about the safety of the bacon.

In 1972, NASA began its use of irradiation to sterilize food for its astronauts when they travelled in space. Scientists and government officials continued their analysis of safety issues, and determined in 1981 that toxicological testing of irradiated food was too insensitive to accurately measure any potential problems. Instead, the FDA created chemical formulas to predict the amounts of irradiated food that could be eaten without showing any noticeable effect on human health.

Opponents of food irradiation technology call it one more threat to food safety, and suggest that it takes attention away from the root causes of the food hygiene problem. They argue that huge farms and industrialized animal agriculture, as well as antibiotics and hormones in animal feed, have contributed to the growing presence of dangerous pathogens in livestock. Irradiation critics challenge the government to clean up the current system of food production, especially in massive slaughterhouses, factory farms, and large-scale food production facilities. These critics also suggest that irradiation may create potentially harmful, resistant bacterial or viral mutants. Finally, they claim that irradiated foods lose a large portion of important vitamins and nutrients during the process, and that they may trigger unexpected allergic reactions in some people.

Food irradiation has been slow to find support in many parts of Europe, especially the United Kingdom. In 2003, a German study prompted the European Commission to place a moratorium on many irradiated foods. In Europe, foods that contain any irradiated ingredients must be labeled and carry the irradiation symbol. In the United States, foods that have been irradiated as a whole must carry the radura label to indicate irradiation, but foods with a mix of irradiated and nonirradiated ingredients do not need a radura label because not all their ingredients are irradiated.

A 2007 proposal by the FDA to modify the way irradiated food is labeled is still being debated by supporters and opponents. The new measure would allow manufacturers to forego a label if they can demonstrate that irradiation does not make material changes to the nutrition or properties of a particular food. The FDA continues to review the proposal, but has no stated timetable for a final decision. At the same time, the FSIS has held hearings on a petition to allow livestock producers to use low-penetration and low-dose irradiation on the surface of chilled beef carcasses without adding the FDA-required radura labels. The FSIS argues that low-dose irradiation would technically be a processing aid and would not, under FDA regulations, require a label. Consumer advocates insist that irradiation labels should be displayed on any treated meat. The FSIS continues to take public comments on the proposal.

In a related move, the FDA increased permissible irradiation levels for fresh iceberg lettuce and fresh spinach. On August 22, 2008, the agency published a new rule that allows the use of a maximum dose of 4 kiloGrays (kGy) of radiation on fresh iceberg lettuce and spinach as well as bagged iceberg lettuce and spinach. The FDA previously allowed those foods to be irradiated at a lower dose to kill insects or slow spoilage. At this time, the packaging of any treated lettuce or spinach must bear the radura logo along with a statement telling consumers it was treated by irradiation. However, agency officials caution that radiation does not replace washing. They recommend that consumers wash all produce before it is eaten unless the packaging specifically states it has been prewashed.

Genetically Modified Organisms

Genetically modified organisms, or GMOs, are considered a food safety issue by some Americans. Supporters see no health risk in GM corn or canola, and support their use in U.S. agriculture. Opponents of GMOs point to a lack of research and suggest they could have hidden dangers for consumers. All known food allergens are proteins, and since genes code for proteins, GM crops end up with a new protein when a foreign gene is inserted. Critics say this could cause unexpected allergic reactions: for example, anyone allergic to fish who eats a tomato that has been genetically modified to include a fish gene could have an allergic reaction to the tomato. Opponents also suggest that, during the process of genetic engineering, the newly inserted gene could damage the plant's own genes or increase the levels of toxins the plant produces.

StarLink corn is an example of what opponents call the impossibility of keeping GM crops separated from their conventional counterparts. In September 2000, U.S. regulators recalled millions of tons of corn and corn-based products after an unapproved strain of genetically modified corn turned up in commercial taco shells. The StarLink corn had only been approved by the FDA for animal feed, not human consumption. However, estimates suggest that more than 50 percent of the U.S. corn supply was contaminated by it that year. Although the company had assured regulators that they could keep StarLink out of the food supply, critics say the incident showed the opposite. After the problem was discovered, two dozen people came forward claiming severe allergic reactions to the StarLink products. The FDA and the CDC conducted tests, and although blood work showed that those people tested had a severe reaction to something, the government determined that StarLink was not the cause.

Opponents of GMOs also question the long-term health effects of eating genetically engineered crops. The most common genetically engineered trait in U.S. corn is Bt-based insect resistance. Bt is short for *Bacillus thuringiensis,* a bacterium that produces toxins that kill insects. Other corn varieties have been engineered to be resistant to certain herbicides or toxic chemicals. Critics argue that there has not been adequate testing on the overall effects of these crops, and that GMOs may eventually have the same serious health impacts as pesticides and other chemical additives—problems that were not discovered until years after many pesticides had been used by consumers.

Recombinant Bovine Growth Hormone

Another controversial technology that has resulted from genetic engineering is the use of bovine growth hormone in dairy cows. Also known as recombinant bovine growth hormone (rBGH) or recombinant bovine somatotropin (rBST), its use in U.S. dairy cows was approved by the FDA in 1993 after years of testing and studies. The hormone, a genetic replica of the hormone the animals produce naturally, was one of the first applications of genetic engineering used in American food production. The hormone is injected into the cows after they give birth, to boost their milk production by up to a gallon per day and keep them making milk longer. The FDA ruled that milk and meat from cows given rBGH were the same as those from other cows and safe for U.S. consumers.

Critics dispute those findings, and warn that rBGH is bad for the health of the cows and may even pose a cancer risk for people. In a 2000 study in the *Journal of Reproductive Medicine,* research showed that women who drank milk with rBGH were three times more likely to have twins than women who did not. The reason appears to be the substance IFG-1 (insulin-like growth factor), which is found in cows' milk and encourages cells to divide. Milk from cows treated with rBGH has three times more IFG-1 than milk from untreated cows. According to the study's author, Dr. Gary Steinman, an assistant clinical professor of obstetrics, his research showed a relationship between bovine growth hormone in the food supply and the fact that the U.S. rate of twin births has almost tripled in the last 30 years.[16] Steinman says the use of assisted reproductive technologies in the U.S. doesn't fully account for the increase in multiple births in this country. He added that "[t]he rate has gone up twice as fast here in the U.S. as in Britain, where there's been a moratorium on synthetic BGH."[17]

Scientific studies have found that high levels of IGF-1 in the blood have been associated with prostate and breast cancer, although no studies have shown that milk from cows treated with rBGH directly causes cancer. Use of the artificial hormone is banned in Canada and the rest of the European Union.

Statistics do show that cows treated with rBGH, sold under Monsanto's brand name Posilac, have higher rates of problems including udder infections, uterine disorders, diarrhea, foot problems, and twin births. Monsanto, the only maker of rBGH in the United States, has maintained for years that there is no difference in milk or dairy products from cows given rBGH. To support that claim, Monsanto sued the Oakhurst Dairy Company of Portland, Maine, in 2003, when that company printed a pledge on its milk containers saying they did not contain artificial growth hormones. Monsanto complained that because they were the only sellers of the hormone for dairy cows in the country, the label must refer to them. Company officials suggested that the label was designed to make milk buyers think there was a difference between milk from cows getting the hormone and other cows, and they argued that this was untrue. The suit was settled when Oakhurst agreed to add the words, "FDA states: No significant difference in milk from cows treated with artificial growth hormone." Monsanto announced in August 2008 that they plan to sell the portion of their business that produces the artificial growth hormone for dairy cows, and to focus instead on their GMO seed and crop business.

CONSUMER GROUPS

Following the *Salmonella* outbreak in the summer of 2008, a number of consumer advocates, scientists, and public health officials called on Congress to reform the FDA via new food safety legislation. With one voice, they asked for a large increase in resources and funding for the FDA, for mandatory recall authority for the FDA and USDA so they could act quickly in public health situations, for traceability in the form of mandated detailed records as a way to follow food all the way back to its origin, and for increased inspections and civil penalties for manufacturers and producers who violate food safety laws. The letter was signed by the Consumers Union, the Consumer Federation of America, the Center for Science in the Public Interest, Public Citizen's Global Trade Watch, the Center for Foodborne Illness Research and Prevention, and Safe Tables Our Priority (STOP).

The Consumer Federation of America is a nonprofit association of some 300 proconsumer groups using research, education, and advocacy to advance the interests of average Americans. The Consumers Union is the nonprofit publisher of *Consumer Reports* magazine; the group's mission, as stated on its Web site, is to advocate a fair, just, and safe marketplace for all U.S. consumers.

The Center for Science in the Public Interest (CSPI) was founded by a small group of scientists during the ecology boom of the early 1970s as an advocate for nutrition, health, and food safety. Characterized as an independent science-based organization, it seeks to educate the public on food and nutrition findings and also to counterbalance the influence of the food industry on government regulations. The organization publishes the award-winning *Nutrition Action Healthletter;* according to the CSPI Web site, this newsletter is considered the largest health publication in North America, with a circulation of 900,000 subscribers. The CSPI is funded by subscriptions to the newsletter and by individual donors. It accepts no advertising, corporate funding, or government grants.

The CSPI celebrated its 35th anniversary in 2006. In 2007, the FDA commissioner awarded the organization the Harvey W. Wiley Special Citation for its work promoting the link between diet and health to consumers, government, and industry. The award is the FDA's highest honor and is named for Dr. Harvey Washington Wiley, an early FDA chief chemist and the first director of what is now the U.S. Department of Agriculture. In 1902, Wiley organized the "poison squad," a volunteer group that tested dangerous chemicals and additives. Wiley was also instrumental in the creation and passage of the 1906 Pure Food and Drugs Act.

The CSPI remains committed to three main goals: providing useful, objective information to the public and to policymakers; representing American consumer interests in developing government regulations; and ensuring that science and technology are used for the public good in connection with research and education for health and nutrition. A recent initiative by the CSPI called for the federal government to require restaurants to display food safety letter grades in their front windows for consumers. The idea started in Los Angeles county restaurants, and is credited by the CSPI with reducing the number of hospitalizations from foodborne illnesses in that area. Las Vegas and St. Louis have adopted similar measures.

Like the CSPI, Public Citizen was founded in the early 1970s as a nonprofit consumer advocacy organization with the specific mission of representing American consumers. Started by Ralph Nader, Public Citizen emphasizes its role as a government watchdog. The organization has six major divisions—Auto Safety, the Energy Program, Global Trade Watch, the Health Research Group, a litigation group, and a division that focuses on Congress—as well as a state office in Texas that was set up in 1984 to focus on global warming and other key environmental issues. Accomplishments listed on Public Citizen's Web site include forcing Red Dye #2 off the market, securing the release of the Nixon White House tapes, and helping to organize massive protests against the World Trade Organization's trade policies. Nader left the group in 1980, and, following his 2000 presidential bid, Public Citizen disassociated itself from him.

The Center for Foodborne Illness Research and Prevention (CFI) is a national nonprofit health organization, started in 2006 by two women whose lives were tragically touched by food poisoning. Executive director Patricia Buck and her daughter, director Barbara Kowalcyk, founded the organization after Kowalcyk's son and Buck's grandson, Kevin Kowalcyk, died from complications due to an *E. coli* infection. Kevin was almost three years old. The organization is dedicated to working with other organizations, the government, and industry to develop better food protections and to prevent foodborne illness through research, education, and advocacy. It is funded through individual contributions, corporate sponsorships, and government grants. Buck volunteered with Safe Tables Our Priority (STOP) before her involvement with CFI. Kowalcyk served as STOP president for two years before founding CFI.

Safe Tables Our Priority (STOP) is another nonprofit organization. It brings attention to the problem of foodborne illness in this country, and describes itself on its Web site as devoted to victim assistance, public education, and policy advocacy for safe food at the grassroots level. The organization started after the 1993 *E. coli* tragedy associated with Jack in the Box hamburgers. Members include scientists, doctors, and people with direct links to the Jack in the Box victims. The organization has three main objectives: it provides information and services to victims of foodborne illness through an information clearing house and hotline; it works to prevent food-related disease outbreaks through public education and media campaigns; and it seeks to reform government and industry practices that permit pathogenic contamination of food from field to table. On its Web site, the group labels itself "a powerful voice for consumers" on food safety policy and regulatory reform at the local and national levels.

FOODBORNE ILLNESS FACTS

Food poisoning is produced by toxins released from bacteria and other organisms when these toxins are eaten. In most cases, this causes stomach cramping, vomiting, diarrhea, and fever, and dehydration when the body loses water faster than it can be replenished. The CDC tracks many of the over 250 foodborne diseases, including infections with the bacteria *Salmonella, Escherichia coli (E. coli), Campylobacter jejuni, Shigella, Listeria*, and *Clostridium botulinum*, and with the Norwalk virus *(Norovirus)*.

The CDC has declared that the most common diseases in America are infections with *Campylobacter, Salmonella, E. coli,* and Norwalk.

Symptoms of *Campylobacter jejuni* infection include diarrhea, cramps, fever, and vomiting. Foods most likely to cause outbreaks include undercooked poultry, unpasteurized or raw milk, and contaminated water. Symptoms usually strike from two to five days after the infected food is eaten, and can last up to 10 days. Researchers suspect that the illness can lead to Guillain-Barré syndrome, a disorder in which the immune system attacks the body's nerves. Early symptoms of Guillain-Barré syndrome include weakness or tingling in the legs that can spread to the arms and upper body. Symptoms can increase in intensity, paralyzing certain muscles. In severe cases, the disorder can be life-threatening. *Campylobacter* has become increasingly resistant to a type of antibiotic used to treat it, and some argue that the overuse of antibiotics in poultry feed has contributed to this development.

Escherichia coli 0157:H7 is one of the several strains of *E. coli* that causes illness. The bacteria brings with it severe diarrhea and often bloody stools along with stomach pain and vomiting, but little or no fever. It can strike anywhere from one day to one week after the bacteria is eaten, and lasts up to 10 days. People with weakened immune systems or children should get medical treatment immediately if they develop symptoms after eating undercooked beef, unpasteurized milk or juice, raw produce, salami, cold cuts, or other deli-style meat and poultry.

Infections with *Salmonella* bacteria mimic the flu, with symptoms that include fever, cramps, muscle aches, vomiting, and diarrhea. Foods suspected of carrying *Salmonella* include eggs, poultry, cheese, raw vegetables and fruit, and unpasteurized milk or juices. The symptoms appear after two or three days, and can last for a week. Severe illness can result if the infection spreads from the intestines to the bloodstream. Some cases have led to organ failure and death.

Listeria monocytogenes can grow slowly at refrigerator temperatures. Symptoms include fever, muscle aches, nausea, and diarrhea. These flu-like symptoms can lead to premature delivery in pregnant women. *Listeria* is often found in fresh soft cheeses, unpasteurized or inadequately pasteurized milk, and deli meats and hot dogs. Gastrointestinal symptoms of may not appear until up to two days after infection, and infections in the blood, brain, or uterus may not appear for two to six weeks. Illness can require immediate medical treatment and can last for months. Of the 2,500 people a year who get seriously sick from *Listeria,* an estimated 500 die.

Shigella bacteria cause the disease shigellosis. Symptoms include diarrhea, fever, and stomach cramps starting a day or two after exposure. A severe infection with high fever may be associated with seizures in children less than two years old. The illness lasts up to a week. People who are infected may not have visible symptoms, but may still pass the bacteria on to others if they do not wash their hands after using the bathroom. Vegetables can be contaminated if they are grown in a field with sewage in it, and flies can breed in infected feces and then contaminate food.

The Norwalk virus *(Norovirus)* differs from other agents of foodborne illness because it is a virus rather than a bacterium. It is often associated with poorly cooked shellfish such as clams and oysters, or with fresh salad ingredients contaminated by infected food handlers. Symptoms include nausea, vomiting, and diarrhea, as well as headache and low grade fever. The CDC estimates that Norwalk virus accounts for up to one-third of the food poisoning cases in the country. A mild and brief illness usually develops one to two days after the contaminated food or water is consumed, and lasts for 24–60 hours. Severe illness or hospitalization is very rare.

Clostridium botulinum is the name of a group of bacteria found in soil that, when exposed to the right conditions, form spores and develop toxins. There are seven types of botulinum toxin designated by the letters A through G; only A, B, E, and F cause illness in humans. Foodborne botulism is often caused by eating home-canned foods with a low acid content, such as asparagus, green beans, beets, or corn. However, there have been reported outbreaks of botulism from unusual sources, such as homemade infused oils or improperly handled baked potatoes wrapped in aluminum foil.

The classic symptoms of botulism include double vision, blurred vision, drooping eyelids, slurred speech, difficulty swallowing, dry mouth, and muscle weakness. To prevent botulism, persons who practice home canning should follow strict hygiene rules, infused oils should be refrigerated, and potatoes baked while wrapped in foil should be kept hot until served or refrigerated. The toxins are destroyed by high temperatures, so boiling food for 10 minutes before eating is a way to ensure the safety of home-canned foods. People who survive an incident of botulism food poisoning can suffer from fatigue or other problems for months to years, and physical therapy may be needed for a full recovery.

Although botulism food poisoning is a rare form of foodborne illness, even more unusual and deadly is mad cow disease. Bovine spongiform encephalopathy (BSE) is a progressive neurological disorder found in cattle. An outbreak of BSE in the 1990s in England was blamed on the practice of feeding British cattle food that contained brains and other parts of infected sheep. To stop the spread of the disease, hundreds of thousands of cows had to be slaughtered. Scientists suspect that the infectious agent is an aberrant protein called a prion, which passes through infected meat and bone meal to young cattle. There is no known cure. Scientific studies have linked variant Creutzfeldt-Jakob disease (vCJD) in humans to BSE. There have been three verified cases of BSE in the United States, the most recent in March of 2006.

New Threats

The infectious and parasitic diseases emerging as new threats to populations all over the world are spread thanks to the increased mobility of people from country to country. The *Cyclospora* parasite is among the almost 30 "new" disease-causing microbes and infectious diseases now recognized by the World Health Organization (WHO). According to the CDC, *Cyclospora* appeared in America in 1996, linked to Guatemalan raspberries. In 2005, health officials blamed *Cyclospora*-contaminated basil for 300 Florida illnesses.

New strains of bacteria, such as *Salmonella* DT104, are starting to show up, and, according to epidemiologists, many of these strains now have a resistance to the drugs most commonly used to treat them. A 1994 outbreak of *Salmonella* DT104 in the United Kingdom killed 10 people. The United States experienced its first outbreak of *Salmonella* DT104 in October 1996. Even familiar strains of *Salmonella* have global significance. *Salmonella enteritidis* infections have increased in 24 of the 35 countries that report outbreaks to the WHO. In the United States, where the infections are linked to the internal contamination of commercial eggs, *Salmonella enteritidis* accounted for 6 percent of reported human infections in 1980, but this figure had jumped to 26 percent by 1994.

Another increasing threat is *E. coli* O157:H7, which was unknown before 1982. Since that time, outbreaks have been reported in Canada, Japan, Africa, the United Kingdom, and the United States. The CDC estimates that there may be about 70,000 infections with *E. coli* O157 in the United States each year. In addition to the bloody diarrhea and other familiar symptoms, *E. coli* O157 has been identified by the CDC as the cause of hemolytic uremic syndrome, a life-threatening complication and the leading cause of kidney failure in American children.

FOOD SAFETY ABCS

Foodborne pathogens are invisible to the naked eye. They don't smell bad or taste funny, but they can make you very sick or even kill you. The newest FSIS education program, the Fight BAC Campaign, was designed to educate consumers on basic food safety. The FSIS lists four cornerstones of food safety: ensure that hands and work surfaces are clean, keep foods separate to prevent cross-contamination, cook to proper temperatures to kill bacteria, and refrigerate food promptly.

Bacteria can spread between countertops, cutting boards, and food so it's important to wash hands and surfaces with hot, soapy water. Anyone handling food should wash his or her hands for at least 20 seconds with warm, soapy water, especially after using the bathroom, changing diapers, handling pets, or touching food. Cloth towels and sponges should be cleaned frequently; cloths should be run through the hot cycle of the washing machine, and sponges through the dishwasher. Produce should also be rinsed under running tap water and scrubbed with a vegetable brush.

Cross-contamination is a serious safety concern when handling raw meat, poultry, seafood, and eggs. The key is to keep these foods away from each other and from the already prepared foods. Cooked food should

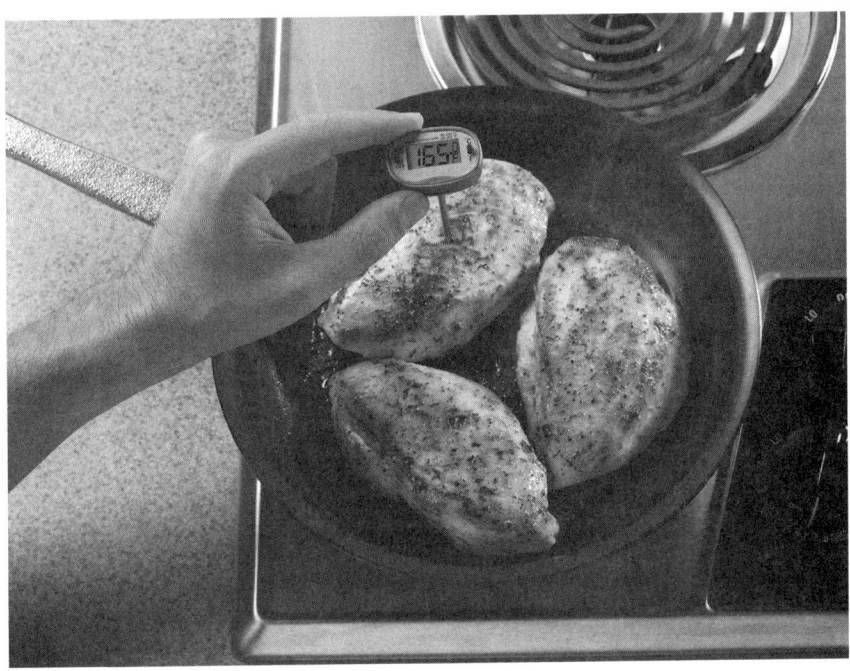

A meat thermometer is an important tool for all home cooks. Meat, like chicken, should be cooked to an internal temperature of 165°F to kill any bacteria. [Courtesy of the USDA Food Safety and Inspection Service]

never be put on a serving plate or cutting board that previously held raw meat, chicken, or seafood without first washing that plate in hot, soapy water. When grocery shopping, consumers should keep meat products, seafood, chicken, and eggs separate from the other foods.

When cooking food, it is difficult to tell by looking whether it has reached a safe minimum internal temperature. Steaks, roasts, and fish need to reach an internal temperature of 145°F, pork; ground beef and egg dishes must reach 160°F; and chicken breasts and whole chickens or turkeys all need to reach 165°F, according to USDA food safety recommendations. Hot dogs, cold cuts, bologna, and other deli meats need to reach a temperature of 165°F when being reheated.

When it comes to leftover food, it is important to refrigerate or freeze meat, chicken, eggs, seafood, or any other perishables within two hours of cooking or purchasing. During the summer, one hour is a safer limit. It is safe to thaw frozen food in the refrigerator, in cold water, or in the microwave, but it is never safe to thaw food at room temperature. Once frozen food is thawed, it should be cooked immediately. The USDA also recommends dividing leftovers into shallow containers for quicker cooling if there is a lot of food to be stored.

There are accepted rules of storage for cooked as well as raw foods. To keep food safe to eat, refrigerator temperatures should not go above 40°F. Eggs can be kept for a maximum of five weeks when fresh, and for one week when hard-boiled. Deli meats that include egg, chicken, ham, and tuna should not be kept more than five days. A package of hot dogs may be refrigerated for a week once opened, and if unopened can be kept for a maximum of two weeks. Ground meats should never be kept in the refrigerator uncooked for more than a day or two, and the same is true for seafood and for chicken or turkey.

Beyond home preparation, shoppers should be careful when buying fresh meat, poultry, and seafood. For example, when buying fresh, whole fish, examine the fish's eyes to be sure they are clear and bulge a little. Only a few fish, such as the walleye, have naturally cloudy eyes. Whole fish or fillets should be firm with shiny flesh. Dull flesh or dark spots around the edges of the fish mean that it is old. The flesh should spring back when pressed, and should have bright red gills free from slime. Any fresh seafood should be used within two days of purchase, and should be kept in the coldest part of the refrigerator or in a special meat-keeper section.

Consumers may be confused by the various types of date labels on food. They include a "Sell-By" date that tells the store how long to display the product for sale; consumers should buy these foods only before the sell-by date. A "Best If Used By" date is only a recommendation; it does not address the safety of the food. A "Use By" date records the last day recommended for the peak quality of the product, as determined by the manufacturer.

THE FUTURE

Foodborne illness is not your grandmother's food poisoning. Today its occurrence, transmission, and control are a serious battleground in a rapidly changing world of pathogens and bacteria. There are as many opinions on how to combat these threats and improve food safety as there are pathogens to make people ill—everything from more regulation to less regulation, from added import fees to no import fees. Unfortunately, the current food safety strategy from both government and industry still puts much of the responsibility on consumer behavior. Their overemphasis on education gives the impression that if people get sick, it is their own fault for not making sure their food was safe. Consumers do have a role to play, but they are only one partner. Government and industry must recognize the importance of safety even if it affects profits.

This is a difficult transition, especially as food prices soar around the globe. The economic reach of the American food industry is enormous. According to FDA figures, the industry contributes more than 20 percent of the U.S. Gross National Product, employs over 14 million Americans, and adds another four million jobs in related industries.[18] The industry's reliance on large, centralized food processing also brings with it an increased risk of larger and more widespread outbreaks of food poisoning, as illustrated by the 1994 outbreak of *Salmonella* from ice cream that sickened 200,000 people in at least 30 states, and by the 2008 *Salmonella* infection of peppers.

If all parties commit to improve agricultural practices, apply food technologies to reduce or eliminate pathogens, and educate persons who handle food, it may be possible to limit the spread of foodborne diseases before they take on larger or more deadly proportions. This will be vital as the U.S. population ages and the number of people with increased susceptibility to these illnesses increases due to higher rates of chronic diseases such as diabetes, heart disease, and hypertension. Also troubling is the shift in the focus of health education in U.S. secondary schools. Health classes now deal primarily with the prevention of alcohol and other drug use, giving little or no attention to food safety education. Is this wise, especially as U.S. eating patterns continue their huge shift to fast-food restaurants and salad bars?

Advocates say the best solution must include regulations and changes in the laws that would keep the pathogens out of the food supply in the first place. Treatments such as irradiation, added antibiotics, or the use of GMOs should not be a substitute for real changes in how government and industry deal with recognized problems. In the end, Americans looking for a reminder of how serious food safety problems can be need only read Upton Sinclair's *The Jungle,* or watch the 1978 cult film, *Attack of the Killer Tomatoes.*

CHAPTER 10

Bans on Fast Food and Junk Food: Who Wins, Who Loses?

It began with a desire for convenience. From the 1950s forward, Americans started cooking less and eating out more. The food changed too: it became fried, processed, and pumped full of salt, fat, sweeteners, and additives. The nation was obsessed with cheap, easy food. Fast-food restaurants multiplied across the country until America had homogenized its landscapes with golden arches, pizza restaurants, taco stands, and burger joints.

By the 1990s, the experience of eating at a fast-food restaurant had become routine. In fact, it is so routine that, according to the National Restaurant Association, Americans spent $134 billion on fast food in 2005 alone. That figure is well above the $110 billion consumers spend yearly on higher education, the $98 billion they spend on new cars, or the $46 billion paid for computer equipment and software.[1] Not only are Americans using more income to eat out, they are eating more meals and spending more on junk food as well. Studies show that the consumption of snack foods has actually doubled in the past 20 years.

Fast-food outlets now encompass everything from hamburgers to tacos, fried chicken, pretzels, cinnamon rolls, cookies, ice cream, and hot dogs. Early pioneers in the fast-food industry included burger restaurants White Castle and McDonald's, and the McDonald's golden arches in particular have reached an iconic status in America. Started in 1948 by the McDonald brothers, Richard and Maurice, McDonald's expanded to 1,000 locations by 1968 and now counts over 31,000 restaurants in 120 different countries. The McDonald's idea was a radical change from the usual diners, sit-down restaurants, or drive-through restaurants, and Richard's building design created one of the most famous corporate logos in the world. The building used two golden arches, lit by neon at night, to form the letter M. It was recognizable from a distance and unique in its design.

Inside the building, the brothers created a service model based on a factory assembly line, with work divided into separate tasks. This new way of doing business solved an ongoing problem with keeping skilled workers. Now, employees only had to be trained for one task. The menu was limited, the food uniform, there was no need for waitresses, and everything was packaged or served in paper wrappers and cups. Historians point to the emergence of this new self-service, fast-food system as the moment when working-class families could afford restaurant food. Junk food, as distinct from fast food, includes pies, cakes, cookies, candy, and sodas. These foods are high in empty calories, are filled with fat and sugar, and lack nutrients, fiber, or protein, and they are sometimes found on fast-food menus in various forms. Even though junk food and fast food are different, both are deeply ingrained in U.S. food culture.

Americans are now seeing the unintended results of their desire for low-priced convenience in the unprecedented numbers of people with obesity, diabetes, and other diseases—brought on at least in part by the American diet high in fat, sweeteners, salt, and additives. Food technologists know that fat, high fructose corn syrup, and sodium are the cheapest ingredients to add flavor to processed food, but their use, especially in fast food, has created an economic paradox.

After reshaping how American families eat, what they eat, and even where they eat it, the food industry is now being asked to improve consumer awareness of nutrition and to offer healthier products. The problem for everyone from candy manufacturers to fast-food restaurants is simple: if they are to stay profitable, they cannot afford to have consumers eat any less of their food. On the other hand, to keep customers happy, manufacturers and restaurants must hold down prices even as officials mandate the use of healthier and costlier ingredients.

For decades, fast-food chains aggressively expanded markets and created new products. Between 1972 and 1995, the U.S. population increased by a third, and the number of fast-food outlets nearly tripled.[2] Fast-food restaurants, soft-drink vending machines, and convenience stores filled with snacks are now on every U.S. corner, putting them within easy reach of all but a few Americans. What happens when the drive to increase profits comes face to face with a growing health crisis of obesity and its related diseases?

In some instances, the government has decided to intervene. Opponents of legislative control compare obesity to tobacco use; antismoking efforts

BANS OF FAST FOOD AND JUNK FOOD

have been legislated for decades with mixed success. Opponents argue that there is still a line between personal responsibility and public health, and that the national focus should be on education and fitness programs. Meanwhile, health advocates hope that laws will force healthy nutrition and convenience to coexist. They argue that government must take action, because the food industry has become so filled with unhealthy food that only legislation can bring balance to the national diet. For America, the outcome is uncertain, but the battle has begun.

LEGISLATIVE ACTION

In September 2008, California Governor Arnold Schwarzenegger signed legislation putting calorie counts on chain restaurant menus and menu boards. Although a similar law had already been passed in 2006 in New York City, this was the first statewide law aimed at improving public health by giving consumers more visible details about their food choices at the

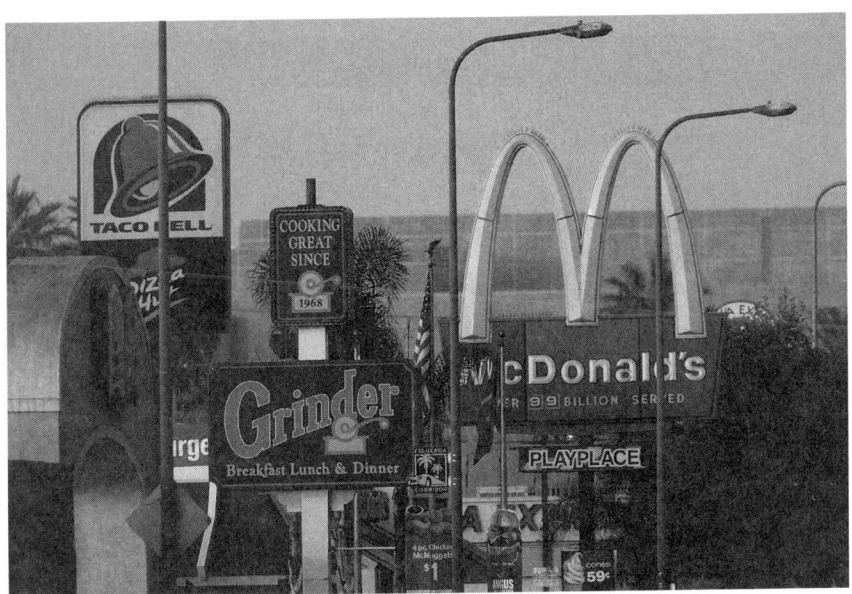

This 32-mile area of South Los Angeles has a greater number of fast-food outlets than neighboring parts of the city, a fact that prompted the city council to initiate a ban. [Getty Images]

point of purchase. The bill allows a phase-in period, and goes into full effect on January 1, 2011. Some 16 other states are considering similar measures, according to a Food Institute report released in October 2008.

On the local level, the Los Angeles City Council passed a fast-food moratorium in the summer of 2008, which stopped any new fast-food or freestanding quick-service restaurants from opening within a 32-square-mile area in the southern part of the city. The one-year moratorium includes two six-month extensions as an option, and is coupled with business incentives to draw more upscale restaurants and grocery stores to the area.

The city council approved the moratorium unanimously after Councilwoman Jan Perry pushed its passage for six years, in an effort to bring what she termed greater food options to the people of South and Southeast Los Angeles. Fast-food restaurants are defined in the ordinance as any restaurant selling food to be eaten on or off the premises with a limited menu of foods made in advance or prepared and heated quickly, offered in disposable wrappers or containers and without table service.

In July 2008, California became the first state in the nation to ban trans fats in all restaurant food as of 2010. Once again, this followed New York City's lead. Similar legislation had been passed in December 2006 by the New York City Board of Health when it voted to ban artificial trans fats from restaurants, school cafeterias, pushcarts, and almost every other food-service operation in the city. Trans fats, or trans fatty acids, are everywhere in the typical American diet. They are created through the hydrogenation process that turns liquid oils into stick margarines or shortening, and are used in cookies, crackers, doughnuts, and many other processed foods.

Food manufacturers turned to trans fats because they increase the shelf life and flavor stability of foods. Unfortunately, studies have shown that, gram for gram, they are more damaging to human health than saturated fat. Not only do trans fats raise levels of the so-called "bad" form of cholesterol, LDL cholesterol, in the body, they also lower "good" HDL cholesterol, thus setting the stage for heart disease. A 2002 consensus report from the National Academy of Sciences Institute of Medicine called the relationship between trans fat consumption and coronary heart disease "linear," and recommended zero trans fats in any diet.[3]

California for years has taken the lead in pushing the public health envelope. In 2004, both the Los Angeles Unified School District and the San Francisco Unified School District implemented bans on soft drinks, candy, and other high-fat snack foods from school vending machines. School districts across the country have followed their lead. The San Francisco policy was tested at one school beginning in January 2003, and school officials noted that food service profits went up after the junk food was removed. Other benefits during the test phase included less litter in the schoolyard, better student behavior after lunch, and elevated school test scores.

The campaign against junk food focused on the advertising front in 2007, when the Center for Science in the Public Interest (CSPI), a consumer advocacy group, filed suit to block advertising for junk foods on shows where 15 percent of the audience is younger than 8 years old. The idea for the suit developed after the release of an Institute of Medicine report, which suggested that there was a direct link between food advertising aimed at children and requests by children for those same high-calorie, low-nutrient foods. As the legislative battle lines continue to be drawn, it is useful to examine the motives and arguments used by government officials as they act to ban fast food and junk food, especially for children.

LEGISLATION PROS AND CONS

The South Los Angeles ordinance is unique because it restricts fast food for public health reasons. The southern part of the city is referred to as a "food desert," a description adopted by social policy planners in the 1990s that describes a growing number of low-income areas with little or no access to affordable, healthy food. Supporters of the LA ban on fast-food restaurants say the law will to attract more full-service restaurants and grocery stories for these neighborhoods, home to mostly black and Hispanic residents, where 28 percent of the people live below the poverty line.

This area of Los Angeles is the birthplace of the Bloods and Crips gangs, and was the epicenter of the 1992 Rodney King riots. Today, among the fading Martin Luther King Jr. murals and the rundown buildings are streets filled with McDonald's, Burger King, Carl's Jr., and Kentucky Fried Chicken restaurants; nearly one out of every two restaurants is a fast-food outlet. Places to buy fresh food are lacking, according to a report by the Community Health Councils (CHC), a local nonprofit agency, which found that there are just 6.8 retail food outlets for every 100,000 residents. That breaks down to one supermarket, grocery, or convenience store for every 6,000 people. This is in stark contrast to nearby West Los Angeles neighborhoods that have 26.6 retail food outlets for every 100,000 residents.[4] People in South Los Angeles who have cars or access to a ride may need to drive 20 minutes or longer to reach full-service national or regional supermarkets, or may spend 45 minutes one way by bus.

Supporters of the fast-food moratorium point to figures from a 2008 study released by the LA County Health Department, which showed that some 30 percent of adults in the affected area were obese, compared with lower obesity rates in other parts of Los Angeles and the nation. Those lower rates ranged from a national average of 21 percent to just over 19 percent for the LA metropolitan area, and 14 percent for the more affluent Westside. Another sobering statistic from the health department report showed a rate of diabetes over 11 percent in South Los Angeles, a figure well above the national average of 8 percent.[5]

Opponents of the controversial law do not dispute those sobering statistics, but they do deride the legislation for "nanny state" tactics designed to stop free enterprise and restrict residents in neighborhoods from making their own decisions about what to eat. They argue that the ban will not affect obesity, does not change the root cause of the problem, and, most importantly, fails to offer education or encourage better eating habits. The answer to the problems, according to these opponents, lies in public education about nutrition, not in using government to stop negative behaviors.

Economist Matthew Turner from the University of Toronto called the ordinance "paternalistic," and suggested that fast-food restaurants dominate that part of Los Angeles because the population wants them there. He pointed out, "If you're a single mother working for minimum wage, you're working 60 hours a week, you need to feed yourself, feed your family. You don't have time to cook so you choose the best thing available, which might be fast food."[6] Opponents recommend that the LA city council focus its attention and resources on fixing the root causes of poverty in that area, or on providing new recreation centers to encourage people to exercise more. They also suggest that even if additional restaurants move into the area, customers may continue to make the same food choices based on price, convenience, and taste.

Fast-food industry representatives also argued against the ban, saying they refuse to accept responsibility if customers choose a double cheeseburger instead of a salad, or a milkshake over a diet soda—especially when the fast-food restaurants already offer a growing list of healthy menu choices. They suggest that the ordinance is part of a larger move to stigmatize fast food, adding that legislation is only necessary in areas where businesses are not profitable or in high crime areas where business owners are afraid of being robbed. According to the CHC, supermarkets have been leaving the South Los Angeles area for the past several years.

There is one encouraging sign. The British grocery retailer, Tesco, has moved into the southwest United States and opened stores in food deserts—a total of 11 stores in Los Angeles and one in South Los Angeles. On the other hand, Whole Foods, which already uses manufacturing and distributing plants in the southern part of Los Angeles, has no plans to open any retail outlets in the area. For now, access to healthy food remains a big problem for low-income Americans. However, history shows that there were other important factors shaping American nutrition.

HISTORY OF PROCESSED FOODS

The proliferation of U.S. fast-food restaurants and limitless supplies of junk food came from a tremendous transformation in twentieth-century America. Born of American ingenuity and fueled by many different factors, the U.S. agriculture industry changed radically in the late-eighteenth and early-nineteenth centuries with the invention of machines and mass production. During the Industrial Revolution, labor-saving machines such as the cotton gin and tractor removed the need for farm labor and pushed an army of rural workers to factory towns to look for work, leaving behind their ability to grow their own food. In a short time, U.S. food production would switch from many small, diversified farms to large, specialized farms that used highly productive methods to yield much larger quantities of food.

Every aspect of American culture was upended by this rapid growth of single-crop agriculture and by the growth of factories and the large urban populations. At the same time, Americans developed greater confidence in processed food, which they were buying in increasing amounts thanks to the passage of the Meat Inspection Act of 1906 and the Pure Food and Drug Act of the same year. By 1920, food processing was the largest industry in the United States, with more earnings than the iron or steel manufacturers.

Transportation also shifted rapidly during this time with the introduction of roads, canals, and railroads. The United States could now ship food hundreds or thousands of miles within its own borders. The arrival of cheap oil further greased the wheels of the fledgling agriculture industry. Before oil and gas flowed into agriculture, farmers had used crop diversity and rotation to replenish the soil, to deal with pests, and to feed themselves, their families, and their neighbors. But cheap gas gave farmers chemical fertilizers, pesticides, and monoculture crops, and offered the ability to ship produce to larger, distant markets.

More changes followed in the aftermath of World War II, when the nation needed to shift from the business of making weapons and munitions. The transfer to fertilizers was easy with ammonium nitrate, the chief ingredient in both chemical fertilizers and bombs. The government also encouraged industry to retool factories that once created nerve gas and other chemical weapons so that they could now make pesticides. Most importantly, the U.S. government subsidized key crops, especially corn and soybeans, and paid farmers to grow as much as they could.

This glut of raw materials became the driving force behind the explosion of animal agriculture. Farms produced abundant grain, which fattened the animals. To increase production numbers, America's meat and dairy animals were moved from the farm to the feedlot. This new ability to mass-produce animal protein led to the availability of plenty of cheap meat and poultry. The days of wartime food rationing were soon forgotten as prosperity spread across the country.

It has always been important for societies to feed their populations. Still, something more important happened with American food policies in this era. Factory towns and cities were filled with people who were working long hours and buying their food from markets, looking for ways to stretch their dollars and reduce time spent cooking meals. Women had entered the workforce during World War II, and continued to be employed in growing numbers. These developments increased the demand for convenience and spurred the trend toward eating out.

The government encouraged farmers to grow corn and soybeans, and those surplus commodities began showing up in all kinds of foods as high-fructose corn syrup and soy oil. The effect of the cheap commodities was to drive down the price of all the food derived from them, including the corn syrup in soft drinks, the soy oil for frying potatoes, and the meat and cheese in burgers.

As food prices went down, American waistlines expanded. There are many reasons U.S. obesity numbers have exploded during the past several decades. The country as a whole settled into a more affluent period, technology made for less physical labor and more sedentary activities, and increasingly effective marketing and advertising encouraged American consumers to buy more and eat more. By the 1960s, fast-food outlets allowed families to pick up food and eat it in their cars or take it home. In fact, food technologists agree that the arrival of fast food, with its convenience and use of sodium, fat, and sweeteners to enhance flavor and texture, was a watershed moment in U.S. nutritional history. The human appetite, with its preference for energy-dense foods high in sugar and fat, could not get enough fries, burgers, nuggets, and sodas.

People have evolved slowly over time, but one thing that has not changed is our taste for these energy-dense foods, thanks to a complicated set of survival mechanisms from our early days as hunters and gatherers. Prehistoric humans needed to build up reserves of fat for lean times or famine. There is also something about human psychology that makes people eat more if it's put in front of them. Americans are fat today because they eat more than is appropriate for their activity level, and their bodies still store excess calories as fat as a protection from starvation.

This increasing mismatch between biology and the environment remains a problem in America because cheap, processed food is so readily available. This phenomenon, known as overnutrition—caused by constant access to heavily processed food—has led to overweight, obesity, and other diseases such as Type II diabetes, heart disease, high blood pressure, and some forms of cancer. According to a report by the United Nations, in the year 2000 the number of people suffering from overnutrition, one billion, had officially surpassed the number suffering from malnutrition, 800 million.[7]

NATIONAL SCHOOL LUNCH PROGRAM

Nowhere is overnutrition more noticeable than among America's youngest citizens. Statistics from the CDC show that obesity rates among children aged 2 to 5 years tripled from 5 percent in the period from 1976 to 1980 to 15 percent from 2003 to 2004. During that same period, obesity figures went from 6.5 percent to almost 19 percent for youngsters aged 6 to 11 years, and jumped from 5 percent to over 17 percent for youths aged 12 to 19 years. According to the CDC, children who are obese are at an increased risk for early onset of heart disease, high blood pressure, diabetes, arthritis-related disabilities, and some cancers.[8]

A new study also found evidence that children who are obese or have high cholesterol are more likely to develop heart disease as they age. Doctors are already seeing an increase in Type II diabetes in children, believed to be a direct consequence of their increased obesity.[9] Ironically, it was the undernourishment of American children that first inspired one of the most significant welfare programs in U.S. history, a program that unfortunately brought fast food and junk food into the daily lives of schoolchildren.

The National School Lunch Program was born out of New Deal politics and signed into law in 1946. From the start, the program linked nutrition to the priorities of agricultural and commercial food interests. During its early years, the number of free lunches served was small, but the program's ability to give farmers an outlet for their surplus commodities was significant. That shifted in the late 1960s and 1970s, when President Richard Nixon dramatically increased funding for the program. He promised during his administration to provide every poor child a free school lunch. In response, Congress increased federal monies for the food, but not for the program's equipment, labor, or operating expenses.

School food directors were caught in a difficult balancing act between cost and nutrition, a conflict that has dogged the school lunch program since the Nixon years and left it conflicted on how to survive financially. To help school lunchrooms serve more free meals and remain economically viable under the new rules, the Department of Agriculture eased restrictions banning commercial operations from school cafeterias. That opened the door to fast-food corporations and giant food service companies.

Over time burgers, fries, pizza, and chicken nuggets made their way into the school lunch program. Schools began feeding children the same high-fat, sugary, salty food during the day that they were often eating at night with their families in fast-food restaurants. These chain restaurants were able to promote their food and to create brand loyalty.

Updated Lunch Laws

School lunches must meet federal nutrition requirements, but the daily decisions about specific foods to serve and how those foods are prepared are left to local school food service directors. Using *Dietary Guidelines for Americans* as a rule of thumb, the food may not have more than 30 percent of its calories as fat, and must contain less than 10 percent as saturated fat. Regulations also establish a standard for school meals to provide one-third of the Dietary Reference Intakes (DRI) of protein, vitamin A, vitamin C, iron, calcium, and calories.

In 1994, the USDA launched the School Meals Initiative for Healthy Children (SMI) to improve the nutritional quality of school meals. Until the SMI, federal nutritional requirements had not changed for almost 50 years, since 1946. As part of the initiative, the USDA published regulations to help schools bring their meals up to date with the Dietary Guidelines.

However, the school programs are required to cook using federally approved commodity foods, many of which are already high in fat. In addition, a report released in 2008 by the Robert Wood Johnson Foundation's Healthy Eating Research showed that more than 50 percent of these commodity foods are sent to processors before they are sent to schools.[10] Processing adds fat, sugar, and sodium. For example, cheese goes on pizza, poultry becomes chicken nuggets, and fruit shows up in a dessert item. The commodity foods that schools must use include frozen ground beef, canned or frozen fruits and vegetables, cheese and cheese products, and rice, pasta, and other grains. The schools are also allowed to use bonus foods over and above entitlement foods, and these come to the schools when there are agricultural surpluses. Bonus foods might include things such as canned sweet potatoes, canned pineapples, or dehydrated potatoes.

Recent findings of the second School Nutrition Dietary Assessment Study (SNDA II) showed that schools are falling far short of meeting

USDA requirements. For starters, meals are too high in fat. The survey for the 1998–1999 school year showed that, on average, 33 percent of calories in elementary school lunches came from fat; only 20 percent of all schools met the guidelines for total fat in the average lunch, and only 14 percent of schools met the guidelines for saturated fat.[11]

Today, schools across the country sell everything from Subway sandwiches to Taco Bell products, Pizza Hut, Domino's, and McDonald's. The American School Food Service Association estimates that about 30 percent of public high schools in the U.S. offer branded fast food. For years, corporate partnerships also brought contracts for soft drink sales into public schools. One Colorado school administrator told the *Denver Post,* "We want kids to think school lunch is a cool thing, the cafeteria a cool place."[12] Those comments eventually became fighting words as parents began to take a hard look at school menus.

Food Fights

Grassroots advocates and moms Susan Rubin and Amy Kalafa were ready for a food fight following the 2007 release of their documentary, *Two Angry Moms,* a film about their parental mission to curb the sale of overly processed, high-sugar foods in U.S. school cafeterias. Kalafa, a veteran independent filmmaker and mother of two, said she was inspired by former Texas Agricultural Secretary Susan Combs, who once said it would take "two million angry moms" to remove all the junk food from school cafeterias and vending machines.

Rubin, a former dentist with a serious interest in nutrition, founded the advocacy group Better School Food in 2005 after she discovered her daughter with candy wrappers from school in her backpack. As a dentist, Rubin was worried about cavities; once she investigated school food, Rubin was even more concerned as a mother about the broader health implications of what school children were eating. That was over 12 years ago, and Rubin's grassroots advocacy group has developed a national following, especially since the release of the documentary.

To make the film, Kalafa followed Rubin and other leaders in the Better School Food movement as they pressed for change. The movie features chefs such as Alice Waters, who successfully reinvented school food in Berkeley, California, with her Edible Schoolyard project. The Edible Schoolyard provides urban public school students with a one-acre organic garden and a kitchen classroom, in an effort to develop their understanding of ecology and nutrition.

The film features several programs over the course of a school year to illustrate how best to connect school cafeterias with classroom learning.

The movie also explores strategies for getting healthy, nutritious food back into school cafeterias. It encourages other parents to step forward and follow the example of these two "fed-up" moms. DVDs and a special information kit to host screenings in homes, schools, or community locations are available for purchase from the Web site www.angrymoms.org.

CONTROLLING PORTION SIZE

It's hard for today's youths to imagine a world without hamburgers and fries, without drive-through service for quick meals, and without grocery store aisles filled with hundreds of brands and flavors of chips and snack foods, or bags full of candy. Without question, the food industry has provided something unique in human history: a dependable, low-cost food supply.

Americans have responded by increasing the volume of food they consume. Marion Nestle, chair of the Department of Nutrition and Food studies at New York University and a nutrition writer, is concerned about the overproduction of food. She notes, "There are 3,800 calories per person per day of food and we only need about half of that."[13] USDA food supply data shows an increase in daily caloric intake by 500 calories per person between 1984 and 2000. On a smaller scale, the USDA data shows an increase of 236 daily calories per person between 1987 and 1995. This minor increase in calories translates into an average 24-pound weight gain every year.[14]

In a country where the word "supersize" is a common verb, and consumers continue to demand more food, snacks, and drinks for their money, it's no surprise that portion sizes are another part of the nutrition problem. For example, in 1957, a fast-food hamburger weighed in at 1 ounce, carrying about 210 calories. Today, a McDonald's Quarter Pounder weighs 6 ounces and provides over 400 calories. The biggest burger on the McDonald's menu is the Double Quarter Pounder with cheese. It tips the scale at 9.8 ounces and 740 calories. In fact, statistics show that every day, one out of fourteen Americans eats at McDonald's—by far the most popular fast-food chain in the world.[15]

In 1977, soda became the most popular beverage in the United States, and Americans now drink some 50 gallons of soda per person per year.[16] The original Coca-Cola bottles contained 6.5 ounces at 79 calories. Now consumers routinely buy 20-ounce containers that provide 250 calories. Many U.S. school districts have dropped their contracts with soft drink makers—and not a moment too soon, in the view of health advocates. According to a report published in the *Journal of the American Heart Association* in July 2007, drinking as little as one can of soda per day—either regular or diet—is associated with an almost 50 percent increase in the risk of heart disease and diabetes and a 30 percent increase in the risk of becoming obese.[17] Officials at the American Beverage Association rejected those study findings as implausible. However, these results and other information continue to provide ammunition for advocates of increasing government bans.

THE CHEESEBURGER BILL

Retailers and food manufacturers cannot wish away sobering health statistics. Although they are trying to reconfigure some products to satisfy critics, their battle remains an uphill one. Many retailers worry that they will eventually be forced to weigh the implications of stocking gourmet ice cream or offering fresh-baked doughnuts against the possibilities of lawsuits. In fact, not everyone in government is anxious to place restrictions on the food industry. Some legislators want to put laws in place to stop legal action against fast-food restaurants and retailers.

The Personal Responsibility in Food Consumption Act was passed by the U.S. House of Representatives in the summer of 2004 to ban obese customers from suing the fast-food chains for making them fat. Nicknamed the "cheeseburger bill," it was an attempt by some legislators to put the responsibility where they believe it belongs—on the individual consumer, not on food manufacturers or restaurants. The bill would not prevent consumers from filing lawsuits if a manufacturer knowingly violated federal and state laws about marketing and labeling food products.

The 2004 effort passed the House, but died a quiet death in the Senate that year for lack of a vote. The legislation was resurrected in 2007 as the Commonsense Consumption Act of 2007 and was introduced in both houses. However, its eventual fate may be a moot point, because some 20 states have already passed similar legislation, and more are expected to follow. Attempts at a national "cheeseburger bill" were prompted by a lawsuit filed in 2002, in which the families of several New York teenagers accused McDonald's of making them fat by serving them highly processed food. U.S. District Court Judge Robert Sweet said in his ruling for the New York lawsuit that "[i]f consumers know or reasonably should know the potential ill health effects of eating at McDonald's, they cannot blame McDonald's if they, nonetheless, choose to satiate their appetite with a surfeit of supersized McDonald's products."[18]

Just what does the average American consumer know about nutrition and healthy food choices? Information is changing in the modern world at breakneck speed. With 24-hour media saturation, this is supposed to be the most informed generation of Americans—which makes it surprising that so many consumers are influenced more by advertising than by hard facts. Perhaps the solution to our national nutrition problem is education, but supporters of legislation to control fast food and junk food consumption are not encouraged by the poor results of earlier attempts to change national tobacco health habits through education. Americans may decide that convenience isn't always the correct choice, and retailers and manufacturers would be wise to take a proactive approach by calling attention to healthy food choices. If government, the food industry, and consumers focus on the simple facts, maybe one day Americans can be led to water (zero calories, zero fat, zero cholesterol, zero sodium) and want to take a drink.

SECTION THREE

References and Resources

APPENDIX A

Annotated Primary Source Documents

I. The Pure Food and Drug Act of 1906 160

II. The DASH (Dietary Approaches to Stop Hypertension)
    Eating Plan 165

III. Guide to the U.S. Food and Drug Administration
     Center for Food Safety and Applied Nutrition (CFSAN)
     Nutrition Facts Label 168

IV. U.S. Department of Health and Human Services
    Amendment to the Food Additives Regulation for
    Irradiation of Eggs... 171

V. U. S. Department of Agriculture Organic Labeling
   and Marketing Information..................................... 176

VI. U.S. Food and Drug Administration Center for Food
    Safety and Applied Nutrition (CFSAN), Excerpted from
    FDA Consumer "The Unwelcome Dinner Guest: Preventing
    Foodborne Illness" 178

VII. The Food and Drug Administration Food Safety and
     Inspection Service (FSIS) Hazard Analysis and Critical
     Control Point (HAACP): A State-of-the-Art Approach to
     Food Safety.. 182

VIII. USDA Food and Nutrition Service National School
      Lunch Program Fact Sheet.................................... 184

IX. Sample Menu for a 2000-Calorie Food Pattern 187

I. THE PURE FOOD AND DRUG ACT OF 1906

The 1906 Pure Food and Drug Act was a landmark document in American history. The act arose in part due to Dr. Harvey Washington Wiley and his work as chief chemist at the Department of Agriculture. Wiley made the study of food adulteration a national issue. Exposés by authors such as Upton Sinclair—who wrote about the meatpacking industry in Chicago—and other muckraking journalists also prompted the enactment of this federal law. The law forbade interstate and foreign commerce in adulterated and misbranded food and drugs. Products found in violation could be seized and condemned, and the responsible person faced fines and jail time. The Pure Food and Drug Act was replaced by a more comprehensive law in 1938.

United States. *United States Statutes at Large* (59th Cong., Sess. I, Chap. 3915, p. 768–772; cited as *34 U.S. Stats. 768*)

AN ACT

For preventing the manufacture, sale, or transportation of adulterated or misbranded or poisonous or deleterious foods, drugs, medicines, and liquors, and for regulating traffic therein, and for other purposes.

Be it enacted by the Senate and House of Representatives of the United States of America in Congress assembled,

SEC. 1. That it shall be unlawful for any person to manufacture within any Territory or the District of Columbia any article of food or drug which is adulterated or misbranded, within the meaning of this Act; and any person who shall violate any of the provisions of this section shall be guilty of a misdemeanor, and for each offense shall, upon conviction thereof, be fined not to exceed five hundred dollars, or shall be sentenced to one year's imprisonment, or both such fine and imprisonment, in the discretion of the court, and for each subsequent offense and conviction thereof shall be fined not less than one thousand dollars or sentenced to one year's imprisonment, or both such fine and imprisonment, in the discretion of the court.

SEC. 2. That the introduction into any State or Territory or the District of Columbia from any other State or Territory or the District of Columbia, or from any foreign country, or shipment to any foreign country of any article of food or drugs which is adulterated or misbranded, within the meaning of this Act, is hereby prohibited; and any person who shall ship or deliver for shipment from any State or Territory or the District of Columbia to any other State or Territory or the District of Columbia, or to a foreign country, or who shall receive in any State or Territory or the District of Columbia, or foreign country, and having so received, shall deliver, in original unbroken packages, for pay or otherwise, or offer to deliver to any other person, any such article so adulterated or misbranded within the meaning of this Act, or any person who shall sell or offer for sale in the District of Columbia or the Territories of the United States any such adulterated or misbranded foods or drugs, or export or offer to export the same to any foreign country, shall be guilty of a misdemeanor, and for such offense be fined not exceeding two hundred dollars for the first offense, and upon conviction for each subsequent offense not exceeding three hundred dollars or be imprisoned not exceeding one year, or both, in the discretion of the court: *Provided,* That no article shall be deemed misbranded or adulterated within the provisions of this Act when intended for export to any foreign country and prepared or packed according to the specifications or directions of the foreign purchaser when no substance is used in the preparation or packing thereof in conflict with the laws of the foreign country to which said article is intended to be shipped; but if said article shall be in fact sold or offered for sale for domestic use or consumption, then this proviso shall not exempt said article from the operation of any of the other provisions of this Act.

SEC. 3. That the Secretary of the Treasury, the Secretary of Agriculture, and the Secretary of Commerce and Labor shall make uniform rules and regulations for carrying out the provisions of this Act, including the collection and examination of specimens of foods and drugs manufactured or offered for sale in the District of Columbia, or in any Territory of the United States, or which shall be offered for sale in unbroken packages in any State other than that in which they shall have been respectively manufactured or produced, or which shall be received from any foreign country, or intended for shipment to any foreign country, which may be submitted for examination by the chief health, food, or drug officer of any State, Territory, or the District of Columbia, or at any domestic or foreign port through which such product is offered for interstate commerce, or for export or import between the United States and any foreign port or country.

SEC. 4. That the examinations of specimens of foods and drugs shall be made in the Bureau of Chemistry of the Department of Agriculture, or under the direction and supervision of such Bureau, for the purpose of determining from such examinations whether such articles are adulterated or misbranded within the meaning of this Act; and if it shall appear from any such examination that any of such specimens is adulterated or misbranded within the meaning of this act, the Secretary of Agriculture shall cause notice thereof to be given to the party from whom such sample was obtained. Any party so notified shall be given an opportunity to be heard, under such rules and regulations as may be prescribed as aforesaid, and if it appears that any of the provisions of this act have been violated by such party, then the Secretary of Agriculture shall at once certify the facts to the proper United States district attorney, with a copy of the results of the analysis or the examination of such article duly authenticated by the analyst or officer making such examination, under the oath of such officer. After judgment of the court, notice shall be given by publication in such manner as may be prescribed by the rules and regulations aforesaid.

SEC. 5. That it shall be the duty of each district attorney to whom the Secretary of Agriculture shall report any violation of this Act, or to whom any health or food or drug officer or agent of any State, Territory, or the District of Columbia shall present satisfactory evidence of any such violation, to cause appropriate proceedings to be commenced and prosecuted in the proper courts of the United States, without delay, for the enforcement of the penalties as in such case herein provided.

SEC. 6. That the term "drug," as used in this Act, shall include all medicines and preparations recognized in the United States Pharmacopoeia or National

Formulary for internal or external use, and any substance or mixture of substances intended to be used for the cure, mitigation, or prevention of disease of either man or other animals. The term "food," as used herein, shall include all articles used for food, drink, confectionery, or condiment by man or other animals, whether simple, mixed, or compound.

SEC. 7. That for the purposes of this Act an article shall be deemed to be adulterated:

In case of drugs:

- *First.* If, when a drug is sold under or by a name recognized in the United States Pharmacopoeia or National Formulary, it differs from the standard of strength, quality, or purity, as determined by the test laid down in the United States Pharmacopoeia or National Formulary official at the time of investigation: *Provided,* That no drug defined in the United States Pharmacopoeia or National Formulary shall be deemed to be adulterated under this provision if the standard of strength, quality, or purity be plainly stated upon the bottle, box, or other container thereof although the standard may differ from that determined by the test laid down in the United States Pharmacopoeia or National Formulary.
- *Second.* If its strength or purity fall below the professed standard or quality under which it is sold.

In the case of confectionery:

If it contains terra alba, barites, talc, chrome yellow, or other mineral substance or poisonous color or flavor, or other ingredient deleterious or detrimental to health, or any vinous, malt, or spirituous liquor or compound or narcotic drug.

In the case of food:

- *First.* If any substance has been mixed and packed with it so as to reduce or lower or injuriously affect its quality or strength.
- *Second.* If any substance has been substituted wholly or in part for the article.
- *Third.* If any valuable constituent of the article has been wholly or in part abstracted.
- *Fourth.* If it be mixed, colored, powdered, coated, or stained in a manner whereby damage or inferiority is concealed.
- *Fifth.* If it contain any added poisonous or other added deleterious ingredient which may render such article injurious to health: *Provided,* That when in the preparation of food products for shipment they are preserved by any external application applied in such manner that the preservative is necessarily removed mechanically, or by maceration in water, or otherwise, and directions for the removal of said preservative shall be printed on the covering or the package, the provisions of this act shall be construed as applying only when said products are ready for consumption.

- *Sixth.* If it consists in whole or in part of a filthy, decomposed, or putrid animal or vegetable substance, or any portion of an animal unfit for food, whether manufactured or not, or if it is the product of a diseased animal, or one that has died otherwise than by slaughter.

SEC. 8. That the term "misbranded," as used herein, shall apply to all drugs, or articles of food, or articles which enter into the composition of food, the package or label of which shall bear any statement, design, or device regarding such article, or the ingredients or substances contained therein which shall be false or misleading in any particular, and to any food or drug product which is falsely branded as the State, Territory, or country in which it is manufactured or produced.

That for the purposes of this Act an article shall also be deemed to be misbranded:

In case of drugs:

- *First.* If it be an imitation of or offered for sale under the name of another article.
- *Second.* If the contents of the package as originally put up shall have been removed, in whole or in part, and other contents shall have been placed in such package, or if the package fail to bear a statement on the label of the quantity or proportion of any alcohol, morphine, opium, cocaine, heroin, alpha or beta eucaine, chloroform, cannabis indica, chloral hydrate, or acetanilide, or any derivative or preparation of any such substances contained therein.
- *Third.* If in package form, and the contents are stated in terms of weight or measure, they are not plainly and correctly stated on the outside of the package.
- *Fourth.* If the package containing it or its label shall bear any statement, design, or device regarding the ingredients or the substances contained therein, which statement, design, or device shall be false or misleading in any particular: *Provided,* That an article of food which does not contain any added poisonous or deleterious ingredients shall not be deemed to be adulterated or misbranded in the following cases:
  - *First.* In the case of mixtures or compounds which may be now or from time to time hereafter known as articles of food, under their own distinctive names, and not an imitation of or offered for sale under the distinctive name of another article, if the name be accompanied on the same label or brand with a statement of the place where said article has been manufactured or produced.
  - *Second.* In the case of articles labeled, branded, or tagged so as to plainly indicate that they are compounds, imitations, or blends, and the word "compound," "imitation," or "blend," as the case may be, is plainly stated on the package in which it is offered for sale: *Provided,* That the term blend as used herein shall be construed to mean a

mixture of like substances, not excluding harmless coloring or flavoring ingredients used for the purpose of coloring and flavoring only: *And provided further,* That nothing in this Act shall be construed as requiring or compelling proprietors or manufacturers of proprietary foods which contain no unwholesome added ingredients to disclose their trade formulas, except in so far as the provisions of this Act may require to secure freedom from adulteration or misbranding.

SEC. 9. That no dealer shall be prosecuted under the provisions of this Act when he can establish a guaranty signed by the wholesaler, jobber, manufacturer, or other party residing in the United States, from whom he purchases such articles, to the effect that the same is not adulterated or misbranded within the meaning of this Act, designating it. Said guaranty, to afford protection, shall contain the name and address of the party or parties making the sale of such articles to such dealer, and in such case said party or parties shall be amenable to the prosecutions, fines, and other penalties which would attach, in due course, to the dealer under the provisions of this Act.

SEC. 10. That any article of food, drug, or liquor that is adulterated or misbranded within the meaning of this Act, and is being transported from one State, Territory, District, or insular possession to another for sale, or, having been transported, remains unloaded, unsold, or in original unbroken packages, or if it be sold or offered for sale in the District of Columbia or the Territories, or insular possessions of the United States, or if it be imported from a foreign country for sale, or if it is intended for export to a foreign country, shall be liable to be proceeded against in any district court of the United States within the district where the same is found, and seized for confiscation by a process of libel for condemnation. And if such article is condemned as being adulterated or misbranded, or of a poisonous or deleterious character, within the meaning of this Act, the same shall be disposed of by destruction or sale, as the said court may direct, and the proceeds thereof, if sold, less the legal costs and charges, shall be paid into the Treasury of the United States, but such goods shall not be sold in any jurisdiction contrary to the provisions of this Act or the laws of that jurisdiction: *Provided, however,* That upon the payment of the costs of such libel proceedings and the execution and delivery of a good and sufficient bond to the effect that such articles shall not be sold or otherwise disposed of contrary to the provisions of this Act, or the laws of any State, Territory, District, or insular possession, the court may by order direct that such articles be delivered to the owner thereof. The proceedings of such libel cases shall conform, as near as may be, to the proceedings in admiralty, except that either party may demand trial by jury of any issue of fact joined in any such case, and all such proceedings shall be at the suit of and in the name of the United States.

SEC. 11. The Secretary of the Treasury shall deliver to the Secretary of Agriculture, upon his request from time to time, samples of foods and drugs which are being imported into the United States or offered for import, giving notice thereof to the owner or consignee, who may appear before the Secretary of Agriculture, and have the right to introduce testimony, and if it appear from the examination of such samples that any article of food or drug offered to be imported into the United States is adulterated or misbranded within the meaning of this Act, or is otherwise dangerous to the health of the people of the United States, or is of a kind forbidden entry into, or forbidden to be sold or restricted in sale in the country in which it is made or from which it is exported, or is otherwise falsely labeled in any respect, the said article shall be refused admission, and the Secretary of the Treasury shall refuse delivery to the consignee and shall cause the destruction of any goods refused delivery which shall not be exported by the consignee within three months from the date of notice of such refusal under such regulations as the Secretary of the Treasury may prescribe: *Provided,* That the Secretary of the Treasury may deliver to the consignee such goods pending examination and decision in the matter on execution of a penal bond for the amount of the full invoice value of such goods, together with the duty thereon, and on refusal to return such goods for any cause to the custody of the Secretary of the Treasury, when demanded, for the purpose of excluding them from the country, or for any other purpose, said consignee shall forfeit the full amount of the bond: *And provided further,* That all charges for storage, cartage, and labor on goods which are refused admission or delivery shall be paid by the owner or consignee, and in default of such payment shall constitute a lien against any future importation made by such owner or consignee.

SEC. 12. That the term "Territory" as used in this Act shall include the insular possessions of the United States. The word "person" as used in this Act shall be construed to import both the plural and the singular, as the case demands, and shall include corporations, companies, societies and associations. When construing and enforcing the provisions of this Act, the act, omission, or failure of any officer, agent, or other person acting for or employed by any corporation, company, society, or association, within the scope of his employment or office, shall in every case be also deemed to be the act, omission, or failure of such corporation, company, society, or association as well as that of the person.

SEC. 13. That this Act shall be in force and effect from and after the first day of January, nineteen hundred and seven. Approved, June 30, 1906.

II. THE DASH EATING PLAN

The 2005 Dietary Guidelines for Americans *provides science-based advice to promote health and to reduce risk for major chronic diseases through diet and physical activity. The intent of the Dietary Guidelines is to enhance the health of most Americans by summarizing and synthesizing knowledge regarding individual nutrients and food components into recommendations for a sensible pattern of eating.*

The DASH (Dietary Approaches to Stop Hypertension) Eating Plan exemplifies the Dietary Guidelines by providing nutrient content estimates for selected foods.

Table A.1 DASH Plan

Food Groups[a]	1,600 Calories	2,000 Calories	2,600 Calories	3,100 Calories	Serving Sizes	Examples and Notes	Significance of Each Food Group to the DASH Eating Plan
Grains[a]	6 servings	6–8 servings	10–11 servings	12–13 servings	1 slice bread 1 oz. dry cereal[b] ½ cup cooked rice, pasta, or cereal	Whole wheat bread, English muffin, pita, bread, bagel, cereals, grits, oatmeal, crackers, unsalted pretzels and popcorn	Major sources of energy and fiber
Vegetables	3–4 servings	4–5 servings	5–6 servings	6 servings	1 cup raw leafy vegetable ½ cup cut-up raw or cooked vegetable ½ cup vegetable juice	Tomatoes, potatoes, carrots, green peas, squash, broccoli, turnip greens, collards, kale, spinach, artichokes, green beans, lima beans, sweet potatoes	Rich sources of potassium, magnesium, and fiber
Fruits	4 servings	4–5 servings	5–6 servings	6 servings	1 medium fruit ¼ cup dried fruit ½ cup fresh, frozen, or canned fruit ½ cup vegetable juice	Apricots, bananas, dates, grapes, oranges, orange juice, grapefruit, grapefruit juice, mangoes, melons, peaches, pineapples, prunes, raisins, strawberries, tangerines	Important sources of potassium, magnesium, and fiber
Fat-free or low-fat milk and milk products	2–3 servings	2–3 servings	3 servings	3–4 servings	1 cup milk 1 cup yogurt 1 ½ oz. cheese	Fat-free or low-fat milk or buttermilk, fat-free or low-fat regular or frozen yogurt, fat-free, low-fat, or reduced-fat cheese	Major sources of calcium and protein

Food group				Serving sizes	Examples and notes	Significance
Lean meats, poultry, and fish	3–4 servings	6 or less servings	6 servings	6–9 servings	1 oz. cooked meats, poultry, or fish 1 egg[c]	Select only lean; trim away visible fats; broil, roast, or boil instead of frying; remove skin from poultry	Rich sources of protein and magnesium
Nuts, seeds, and legumes	3–4 servings/week	4–5 servings/week	1 serving	1 serving	⅓ cup or 1½ oz. nuts 2 Tbsp peanut butter 2 Tbsp or ½ oz. seeds ½ cup cooked dry beans or peas	Almonds, filberts, mixed nuts, peanuts, walnuts, sunflower seeds, kidney beans, lentils	Rich sources of energy, magnesium, potassium, protein, and fiber
Fats and oils[d]	2 servings	2–3 servings	3 servings	4 servings	1 tsp soft margarine 1 Tbsp mayonnaise 2 Tbsp salad dressing 1 tsp vegetable oil	Soft margarine, low-fat mayonnaise, light salad dressing, vegetable oil (such as olive, corn, canola, or safflower)	The DASH study had 27 percent of calories as fat (low in saturated fat), including fat in or added to foods
Sweets	0 servings	5 or less servings/week	2 or less servings	2 or less servings	1 Tbsp sugar 1 Tbsp jelly or jam ½ cup sorbet and ices 1 cup lemonade	Maple syrup, sugar, jelly jam, fruit-flavored gelatin, hard candy, fruit punch, sorbet and ices	Sweets should be low in fat

[a] Whole grains are recommended for most grain servings to meet fiber recommendations.
[b] Equals 1/2 cup to 1 1/4 cups, depending on cereal type. Check the product's Nutrition Facts label.
[c] Since eggs are high in cholesterol, limit egg yolk intake to no more than four per week; two egg whites have the same protein content as 1 oz of meat.
[d] Fat content changes serving amount for fats and oils. For example, 1 Tbsp of regular salad dressing equals one serving; 1 Tbsp of a low-fat dressing equals one-half serving; 1 Tbsp of a fat-free dressing equals zero servings.

Abbreviations: oz = ounce; Tbsp = tablespoon; tsp = teaspoon.

[Courtesy of the U.S. Department of Agriculture]

Originally developed to study the effects of an eating pattern on the prevention and treatment of hypertension, the DASH plan now presents a sample seven-day menu consistent with the 2005 Dietary Guidelines.

The DASH Eating Plan offers menus for a variety of calorie levels, recognizing that recommended calorie intake will differ for individuals based on age, gender, and activity level. At each calorie level, individuals who eat nutrient-dense foods may be able to meet their recommended nutrient intake without consuming their full calorie allotment. The remaining calories—the discretionary calorie allowance—allow individuals flexibility to consume some foods and beverages that may contain added fats, added sugars, and alcohol. The recommendations in the Dietary Guidelines are for Americans over two years of age. The DASH Eating Plan is flexible enough to accommodate a range of food preferences and cuisines, and can also incorporate the food preferences of different racial/ethnic populations, vegetarians, and other groups.

The DASH eating plan is based on 1,600, 2,000, 2,600 and 3,100 calories. The number of daily servings in a food group var[ies] depending on caloric needs. This chart can aid in planning menus and food selection in restaurants and grocery stores.

Note: Table updated to reflect 2006 DASH Eating Plan.

III. CFSAN's Guide to the Nutrition Facts Label

The U.S. Food and Drug Administration Center for Food Safety and Applied Nutrition (CFSAN) is responsible for creating information to educate consumers about labeling requirements under the Federal Food, Drug, and Cosmetic Act and its amendments. Food labeling is mandatory for most prepared foods, such as breads, cereals, canned and frozen foods, snacks, desserts, drinks, and so on. The Nutrition Facts Label for such foods contains detailed information designed to provide specifics on calories, fats, vitamins, minerals, and other recommended dietary information. A detailed explanation from the CFSAN, excerpted below, offers a step-by-step overview of the label components.

The Nutrition Facts Label—An Overview

The information in the main or top section (see #1–4 and #6 on the sample nutrition label below), can vary with each food product; it contains product-specific information (serving size, calories, and nutrient information). The bottom part (see #5 on the sample label below) contains a footnote with Daily Values (DVs) for 2,000 and 2,500 calorie diets. This footnote provides recommended dietary information for important nutrients, including fats, sodium and fiber. The footnote is found only on larger packages and does not change from product to product.

Courtesy of the U. S. Food and Drug Administration Center for Food Safety and Applied Nutrition

ANNOTATED PRIMARY SOURCE DOCUMENTS

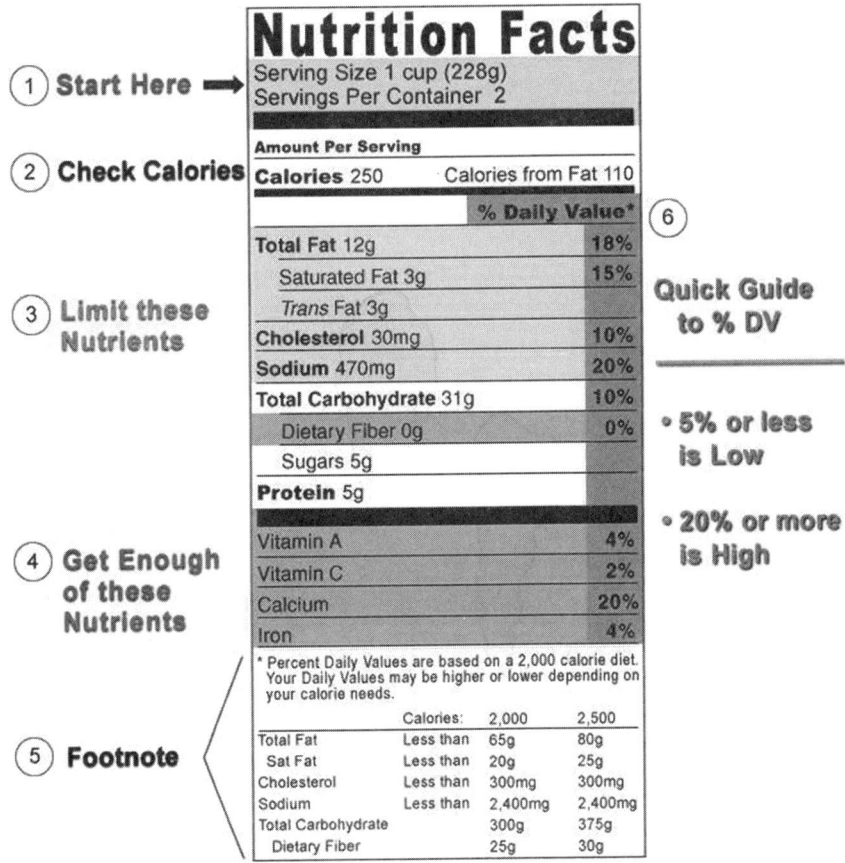

[Courtesy of the U. S. Food and Drug Administration Center for Food Safety and Applied Nutrition]

1. The Serving Size

The first place to start when you look at the Nutrition Facts label is the serving size and the number of servings in the package. Serving sizes are standardized to make it easier to compare similar foods; they are provided in familiar units, such as cups or pieces, followed by the metric amount, e.g., the number of grams.

The size of the serving on the food package influences the number of calories and all the nutrient amounts listed on the top part of the label. Pay attention to the serving size, especially how many servings there are in the food package. Then ask yourself, "How many servings am I consuming?" (e.g., 1/2 serving, 1 serving, or more). In the sample label, one serving of macaroni and cheese equals one cup. If you ate the whole package, you would eat two cups. That doubles the calories and other nutrient numbers, including the % Daily Values as shown in the sample label.

2. Calories (and Calories from Fat)

Calories provide a measure of how much energy you get from a serving of this food. Many Americans consume more calories than they need without meeting recommended intakes for a number of nutrients. The calorie section of the label can help you manage your weight (i.e., gain, lose, or maintain.) Remember: the number of servings you consume determines the number of calories you actually eat (your portion amount).

In the example, there are 250 calories in one serving of this macaroni and cheese. How many calories from fat are there in ONE serving? Answer: 110 calories, which means almost half the calories in a single serving come from fat. What if you ate the whole package content? Then, you would consume two servings, or 500 calories, and 220 would come from fat.

The General Guide to Calories provides a general reference for calories when you look at a Nutrition Facts label. This guide is based on a 2,000 calorie diet. Eating too many calories per day is linked to overweight and obesity.

3, 4. The Nutrients: How Much?

Look at the top of the nutrient section in the sample label. It shows you some key nutrients that impact on your health and separates them into two main groups: The nutrients listed first are the ones Americans generally eat in adequate amounts, or even too much. They are identified in yellow as "Limit These Nutrients." Eating too much fat, saturated fat, trans fat, cholesterol, or sodium may increase your risk of certain chronic diseases, like heart disease, some cancers, or high blood pressure. Important: Health experts recommend that you keep your intake of saturated fat, trans fat and cholesterol as low as possible as part of a nutritionally balanced diet.

Most Americans don't get enough dietary fiber, vitamin A, vitamin C, calcium, and iron in their diets. They are identified in blue as "Get Enough of These Nutrients." Eating enough of these nutrients can improve your health and help reduce the risk of some diseases and conditions. For example, getting enough calcium may reduce the risk of osteoporosis, a condition that results in brittle bones as one ages. Eating a diet high in dietary fiber promotes healthy bowel function. Additionally, a diet rich in fruits, vegetables, and grain products that contain dietary fiber, particularly soluble fiber, and low in saturated fat and cholesterol may reduce the risk of heart disease.

Remember: You can use the Nutrition Facts label not only to help *limit* those nutrients you want to cut back on but also to *increase* those nutrients you need to consume in greater amounts.

5. Understanding the Footnote on the Bottom of the Nutrition Facts Label

Note the * used after the heading "% Daily Value" on the Nutrition Facts label. It refers to the Footnote in the lower part of the nutrition label, which tells you "%DVs are based on a 2,000-calorie diet." This statement must be on all food labels. But the remaining information in the full footnote may not be on the package if the size of the label is too small. When the full footnote does appear, it will always be the same. It doesn't change from product to product, because it shows recommended dietary advice for all Americans—it is not about a specific food product.

6. The Percent Daily Value (%DV)

The % Daily Values (%DVs) are based on the Daily Value recommendations for key nutrients but only for a 2,000 calorie daily diet—not 2,500 calories. You, like most people, may not know how many calories you consume in a day. But you can still use the %DV as a frame of reference whether or not you consume more or less than 2,000 calories.

IV. AMENDMENT TO THE FOOD ADDITIVES REGULATION FOR IRRADIATION OF EGGS

The U.S. Department of Health and Human Services oversees the Food and Drug Administration (FDA) and its rules governing the use of ionizing radiation in U.S. food production. As additional food items were approved for radiation, the FDA continued to amend these regulations. In 1998, the FDA received a petition proposing that food additive regulations concerning part 179 (Irradiation in the Production, Processing and Handling of Food) be amended to include treatment of fresh shell eggs to reduce Salmonella. *The approved changes became effective on July 21, 2000.*

DEPARTMENT OF HEALTH AND HUMAN SERVICES
Food and Drug Administration
21 CFR Part 179
[Docket No. 98F-0165]
Irradiation in the Production, Processing and Handling of Food
AGENCY: Food and Drug Administration, HHS.
ACTION: Final rule.
SUMMARY: The Food and Drug Administration (FDA) is amending the food additive regulations to provide for the safe use of ionizing radiation for the reduction of *Salmonella* in fresh shell eggs. This action is in response to a petition filed by Edward S. Josephson.
DATES: This rule is effective July 21, 2000. Submit written objections and requests for a hearing by August 21, 2000.
ADDRESSES: Submit written objections to the Dockets Management Branch (HFA-305), Food and Drug Administration, 5630 Fishers Lane, rm. 1061, Rockville, MD 20852.
FOR FURTHER INFORMATION CONTACT: William J. Trotter, Center for Food Safety and Applied Nutrition (HFS-206), Food and Drug Administration, 200 C St. SW, Washington, DC 20204, 202-418-3088.
SUPPLEMENTARY INFORMATION:

I. Background

In a notice published in the Federal Register of March 20, 1998 (63 FR 13675), FDA announced that a food additive petition (FAP 8M4584) had been filed by Edward S. Josephson, University of Rhode Island, Food Science and Nutrition Research Center, 530 Liberty Lane, West Kingston, RI 02892-1802. The petitioner proposed that the food additive regulations in part 179, Irradiation in the Production, Processing and Handling of Food (21 CFR part 179), be amended to provide for the safe use of ionizing radiation for the reduction of *Salmonella* in fresh shell eggs.

II. Safety Evaluation

Under section 201(s) of the Federal Food, Drug, and Cosmetic Act (the act) (21 U.S.C. 321(s)), a source of radiation used to treat food is defined as a food additive. The additive is not, literally, added to food. Instead, a source of radiation is used to process or treat food such that, analogous to other food processes, its use can affect the characteristics of the food. In the subject petition, the intended technical effect is a change in the microbial load of the food, specifically, a reduction in the numbers of *Salmonella*, a human pathogen, in or on fresh shell eggs.

The petitioner submitted published articles and other study reports containing data and information related to eggs and other kinds of food in the areas of radiation chemistry, nutrition, toxicology, and microbiology. FDA has fully considered the data and studies submitted in the petition, as well as other information in its files relevant to the safety and nutritional adequacy of eggs treated with ionizing radiation.

The effects of ionizing radiation on the characteristics of treated foods are a direct result of the chemical reactions induced by the absorbed radiation. Scientists have compiled a large body of data regarding the effects of ionizing radiation on different foods under various conditions of irradiation. Research has established that the types and amounts of products generated by radiation-induced chemical reactions (hereinafter referred to as "radiolysis products") depend on the chemical constituents of the food and on the conditions of irradiation (e.g., temperature and presence or absence of air and moisture). Furthermore, the principles of radiation chemistry govern the extent of changes both in the nutrient levels and in the microbial load of irradiated foods. Key factors include the specific nutrient or microorganism of interest, the food, and the conditions of irradiation. (See the agency's final rule permitting the irradiation of meat (the meat final rule) in the Federal Register of December 3, 1997 (62 FR 64107) for FDA's discussion of radiation chemistry, nutrition, toxicology, and microbiology related to irradiation of foods composed primarily of water, protein, and lipids under various conditions of irradiation.)

FDA has reviewed the relevant data and information submitted in the petition regarding the radiation chemistry of fresh shell eggs, and data available in the agency's files. Fresh whole eggs are composed mainly of water (75.3 percent), protein (12.5 percent), and lipid (10.0 percent) (Ref. 1). As discussed in the meat final rule, the radiation chemistry associated with these types of compounds is well known. FDA has concluded that the concentrations and types of radiolysis products formed by the irradiation of eggs will be comparable to those products produced by the irradiation of other foods of similar composition, such as meat (Ref. 2). In addition, the petitioner's data support the conclusion that there is little change in the levels of individual fatty acids, or in the structure, digestibility, or biological value of protein, when shell eggs are treated with ionizing radiation up to 3 kiloGray (kGy) (Refs. 2 and 3). Most of the radiolysis products are either the same as, or structurally similar to, compounds found in foods that have not been irradiated, and are formed in very small amounts. In summary, an absorbed dose of 3 kGy for the irradiation of fresh shell eggs will result in only minimal changes in the macronutrients (protein, lipid, or carbohydrate), and the chemical composition of eggs will not differ in any significant manner from eggs that have not been irradiated.

The petitioner submitted studies and published reports relevant to the safety of irradiated foods, in general. In addition, a variety of irradiated foods including: Red meat, chicken, fish, and eggs, have been tested in earlier animal feeding studies and genotoxicity studies; and they were previously reviewed by FDA (see, e.g., 62 FR 64107, December 3, 1997). Included in the information considered by FDA in the review of this petition are three studies conducted specifically on irradiated eggs (Ref. 4). In the first such study, rats were fed a biscuit diet containing whole eggs irradiated at 5 kGy at a dietary level of 25 percent on a dry weight basis for 3 years (two generations). No adverse effects were observed compared to the control group fed a diet containing nonirradiated eggs. In the second study, mice and rats were fed a diet containing dried eggs irradiated at 93 kGy and irradiated pork brain. No effects were observed that were attributed to the irradiated food. In the third study, rats were fed canned eggs irradiated at 5 kGy in their diet for two generations. No effects were observed that were attributed to the irradiated diet. Taken as a whole, based on the totality of evidence from all evaluated data and studies, FDA concludes that the petitioned use of irradiation on fresh shell eggs raises no toxicity concerns (Refs. 4 and 5).

FDA also evaluated the effects of irradiation processing on micronutrients (e.g., minerals, water-soluble vitamins, and fat-soluble vitamins). Minerals are unaffected by irradiation, but the levels of some vitamins may be reduced as a result of irradiation. For example, vitamin A levels did decrease with an increasing radiation dose. Not all vitamin loss is significant, however. The extent to which a reduction in a specific vitamin level is significant depends on the relative contribution from the food in question to the dietary intake of the vitamin and the overall sufficiency of the vitamin in the diet. Based upon data in the agency's files, FDA concludes that the intake of vitamins from other foods compensates for the vitamin loss from the irradiation of eggs (Refs. 4 and 5). For example, a fresh unirradiated egg contains approximately 95 retinol equivalents (RE) of vitamin A (Ref. 4). In a study, shell eggs irradiated at 1.0 kGy and stored for 24 days contained approximately 72 RE's (Ref. 3). In comparison, 1 tablespoon of butter contains 108 RE's, one-half cup of bran cereal contains 258 RE's, and one-half cup of canned carrots contains 1,620 RE's of vitamin A (Ref. 4). FDA, therefore, concludes, based upon all the evidence before it, that irradiation of fresh shell eggs under the conditions set forth in the regulation below will not have an adverse impact on the nutritional adequacy of a person's diet.

Increased irradiation levels can also cause organoleptic changes in the egg. For example, data in the petition showed an increased color loss in the irradiated egg yolk and a change in the egg's viscosity as the radiation dose was increased. Thus, FDA expects that the acceptability of irradiated shell eggs, based on their color and viscosity, will limit, in a practical way, the maximum dose of irradiation applied to fresh shell eggs. Therefore, FDA has determined that there is no need to limit the irradiation level based on changes in micronutrient levels or organoleptic characteristics of the eggs.

Irradiation of fresh shell eggs at the doses requested in the petition will reduce, but not entirely eliminate, microorganisms in eggs. The stated purpose of this petition is for approval of radiation of fresh shell eggs to reduce the number of *Salmonella*. The data show that low dose irradiation in the range requested by the petitioner can reduce the levels of *S. enteritidis* in fresh shell eggs (Ref. 6). *Salmonella* strains, in addition to *S. enteritidis*, in fresh shell eggs should also be reduced by irradiation since *S. enteritidis* was found to have similar sensitivities to ionizing radiation as five other strains of *Salmonella* that were tested in various media (Ref. 7).

Based on the data and studies submitted in the petition and other information in the agency's files, FDA concludes that: (1) The proposed use of irradiation on fresh shell eggs at levels not to exceed 3.0 kGy is safe, (2) the irradiation can achieve its intended technical effect and, therefore, (3) the regulations in Sec. 179.26 (21 CFR 179.26) should be amended as set forth below.

In accordance with Sec. 171.1(h) (21 CFR 171.1(h)), the petition and the documents that FDA considered and relied upon in reaching its decision to approve the petition are available for inspection at the Center for Food Safety and Applied Nutrition by appointment with the information contact person listed above. As provided in Sec. 171.1(h), the agency will delete from the documents any materials that are not available for public disclosure before making the documents available for inspection.

This final rule contains no collections of information. Therefore, clearance by the Office of Management and Budget under the Paperwork Reduction Act of 1995 is not required.

III. Environmental Impact

The agency has previously considered the environmental effects of this rule as announced in the filing notice for FAP 8M4584 (63 FR 13675, March 20, 1998). No new information or comments have been received that would affect the agency's previous determination that there is no significant impact on the human environment and that an environmental impact statement is not required.

IV. Objections

Any person who will be adversely affected by this regulation may at any time file with the Dockets Management Branch (address above) written objections by

August 21, 2000. Each objection shall be separately numbered, and each numbered objection shall specify with particularity the provisions of the regulation to which objection is made and the grounds for the objection. Each numbered objection on which a hearing is requested shall specifically so state. Failure to request a hearing for any particular objection shall constitute a waiver of the right to a hearing on that objection. Each numbered objection for which a hearing is requested shall include a detailed description and analysis of the specific factual information intended to be presented in support of the objection in the event that a hearing is held. Failure to include such a description and analysis for any particular objection shall constitute a waiver of the right to a hearing on the objection. Three copies of all documents are to be submitted and are to be identified with the docket number found in brackets in the heading of this document. Any objections received in response to the regulation may be seen in the Dockets Management Branch between 9 a.m. and 4 p.m., Monday through Friday.

V. References

The following references have been placed on display at the Dockets Management Branch (address above) and may be seen by interested persons between 9 a.m. and 4 p.m., Monday through Friday.

1. Nutrient Data Laboratory Food Composition Data, USDA Agricultural Research Service, available at Internet address: http://www.nal.usda.gov/fnic/foodcomp.
2. Memorandum from K. Morehouse, FDA, to W. Trotter, FDA, May 14, 1999.
3. Memorandum from K. Morehouse, FDA, to W. Trotter, FDA, April 11, 2000.
4. Memorandum from I. Chen, FDA, to W. J. Trotter, FDA, December 11, 1998.
5. Memorandum from I. Chen, FDA, to W. J. Trotter, FDA, March 31, 2000.
6. Memorandum from V. K. Bunning, FDA, to W. J. Trotter, FDA, April 4, 2000.
7. Thayer, D.W., et al., "Radiation Resistance of *Salmonella*," Journal of Industrial Microbiology, 5:383–390, 1990.

List of Subjects in 21 CFR Part 179

Food additives, Food labeling, Food packaging, Radiation protection, Reporting and recordkeeping requirements, Signs and symbols.

Final Action Taken

Therefore, under the Federal Food, Drug, and Cosmetic Act and under authority delegated to the Commissioner of Food and Drugs and redelegated to the Director, Center for Food Safety and Applied Nutrition, 21 CFR part 179 is amended as follows:

PART 179—IRRADIATION IN THE PRODUCTION, PROCESSING AND HANDLING OF FOOD

1. The authority citation for 21 CFR part 179 continues to read as follows: Authority: 21 U.S.C. 321, 342, 343, 348, 373, 374.

2. Section 179.26 is amended in the table in paragraph (b) by adding entry "9." under the headings "Use" and "Limitations" to read as follows:

Sec. 179.26 Ionizing radiation for the treatment of food.

Use	Limitations
9. For control of *Salmonella* in fresh shell eggs.	Not to exceed 3.0 kGy.

Dated: July 14, 2000.
L. Robert Lake,
Director of Regulations and Policy, Center for Food Safety and Applied Nutrition.
[FR Doc. 00-18496 Filed 7-20-00; 8:45 am]
BILLING CODE 4160-01-F
FDA/Center for Food Safety & Applied Nutrition

V. USDA's Organic Labeling and Marketing Information

The U.S. Department of Agriculture (USDA) administers the National Organic Program (NOP), the federal regulatory framework governing organic food in the United States. Under the NOP, farmers and food processors using the word "organic" on their packaging or labeling information must be certified, based on national standards for organic products developed following passage of the Organic Food Production Act of 1990. This USDA Agricultural Marketing Service (AMS) document (October 2002; updated April 2008) details the NOP labeling requirements, and other provisions and penalties.

The Organic Foods Production Act (OFPA) and the National Organic Program (NOP) assure consumers that the organic agricultural products they purchase are produced, processed, and certified to consistent national organic standards. The labeling requirements of the NOP apply to raw, fresh products and processed products that contain organic agricultural ingredients. Agricultural products that are sold, labeled, or represented as organic must be produced and processed in accordance with the NOP standards.

Except for operations whose gross income from organic sales totals $5,000 or less, farm and processing operations that grow and process organic agricultural products must be certified by USDA-accredited certifying agents.

Labeling requirements are based on the percentage of organic ingredients in a product.

Agricultural Products Labeled "100 Percent Organic" and "Organic"

Products labeled as "100 percent organic" must contain (excluding water and salt) only organically produced ingredients and processing aids.

Products labeled "organic" must consist of at least 95 percent organically produced ingredients (excluding water and salt). Any remaining product ingredients must consist of nonagricultural substances approved on the National List including specific non-organically produced agricultural products that are not commercially available in organic form.

Products meeting the requirements for "100 percent organic" and "organic" may display these terms and the percentage of organic content on their principal display panel.

The USDA seal and the seal or mark of involved certifying agents may appear on product packages and in advertisements.

Agricultural products labeled "100 percent organic" and "organic" cannot be produced using excluded methods, sewage sludge, or ionizing radiation.

Processed Products Labeled "made with Organic Ingredients"

Processed products that contain at least 70 percent organic ingredients can use the phrase "made with organic ingredients" and list up to three of the organic ingredients or food groups on the principal display panel. For example, soup made with at least 70 percent organic ingredients and only organic vegetables may be labeled either "soup made with organic peas, potatoes, and carrots," or "soup made with organic vegetables."

Processed products labeled "made with organic ingredients" cannot be produced using excluded methods, sewage sludge, or ionizing radiation. The percentage of organic content and the certifying agent seal or mark may be used on the principal display panel. However, the USDA seal cannot be used anywhere on the package.

Processed Products that Contain Less than 70 Percent Organic Ingredients

These products cannot use the term organic anywhere on the principal display panel. However, they may identify the specific ingredients that are organically produced on the ingredients statement on the information panel.

Other Labeling Provisions

Any product labeled as organic must identify each organically produced ingredient in the ingredient statement on the information panel.

The name of the certifying agent of the final product must be displayed on the information panel. The address of the certifying agent of the final product may be displayed on the information panel.

There are no restrictions on use of other truthful labeling claims such as "no drugs or growth hormones used," "free range," or "sustainably harvested."

Penalties for Misuse of Labels

A civil penalty of up to $11,000 can be levied on any person who knowingly sells or labels as organic a product that is not produced and handled in accordance with the National Organic Program's regulations.

VI. CFSAN's Preventing Foodborne Illness

The U.S. Food and Drug Administration Center for Food Safety and Applied Nutrition (CFSAN) creates consumer advice publications on food safety, nutrition, and cosmetics. Those question and answer sheets include tips on topics including foodborne illness, food storage, food preparation, nutrition, dietary supplements, and weight loss. These tips are excerpted from FDA Consumer, *"The Unwelcome Dinner Guest: Preventing Foodborne Illness" (Jan.-Feb. 1991; revised Dec. 1997, Feb. 1999, Oct. 1999, June 2000, July 2002, and March 2003).*

Prevention Tips

The idea that the food on the dinner table can make someone sick may be disturbing, but there are many steps you can take to protect your families and dinner guests. It's just a matter of following basic rules of food safety.

Prevention of foodborne illness starts with your trip to the supermarket.

- Pick up your packaged and canned foods first.
- Don't buy food in cans that are bulging or dented or in jars that are cracked or have loose or bulging lids.
    Don't eat raw shellfish, and use only pasteurized milk and cheese and pasteurized or otherwise treated ciders and juices if you have a health problem, especially one that may have impaired your immune system.
- Choose eggs that are refrigerated in the store. Before putting them in your cart, open the carton and make sure that the eggs are clean and none are cracked.
- Select frozen foods and perishables such as meat, poultry or fish last. Always put these products in separate plastic bags so that drippings don't contaminate other foods in your shopping cart.
- Don't buy frozen seafood if the packages are open, torn or crushed on the edges. Avoid packages that are above the frost line in the store's freezer. If the package cover is transparent, look for signs of frost or ice crystals. This could mean that the fish has either been stored for a long time or thawed and refrozen.
- Check for cleanliness at the meat or fish counter and the salad bar. For instance, cooked shrimp lying on the same bed of ice as raw fish could become contaminated.
- When shopping for shellfish, buy from markets that get their supplies from state-approved sources; stay clear of vendors who sell shellfish from roadside stands or the back of a truck. And if you're planning to harvest your own shellfish, heed posted warnings about the safety of the water.
- Take an ice chest along to keep frozen and perishable foods cold if it will take more than an hour to get your groceries home.

Safe Storage

- The first rule of food storage in the home is to refrigerate or freeze perishables right away. The refrigerator temperature should be 40 degrees Fahrenheit (5 degrees Celsius), and the freezer should be zero [degrees] F (minus 18°C). Check both "fridge" and freezer periodically with a refrigerator/freezer thermometer.
- Poultry and meat heading for the refrigerator may be stored as purchased in the plastic wrap for a day or two. If only part of the meat or poultry is going to be used right away, it can be wrapped loosely for refrigerator storage. Just make sure juices can't escape to contaminate other foods.
- Wrap tightly foods destined for the freezer. Leftovers should be stored in tight containers.
- Store eggs in their carton in the refrigerator itself rather than on the door, where the temperature is warmer.
- Seafood should always be kept in the refrigerator or freezer until preparation time.
- Don't crowd the refrigerator or freezer so tightly that air can't circulate. Check the leftovers in covered dishes and storage bags daily for spoilage. Anything that looks or smells suspicious should be thrown out.
- A sure sign of spoilage is the presence of mold, which can grow even under refrigeration. While not a major health threat, mold can make food unappetizing. Most moldy foods should be thrown out. But you might be able to save molding hard cheeses, salami, and firm fruits and vegetables if you cut out not only the mold but a large area around it. Cutting the larger area around the mold is important because much of the mold growth is below the surface of the food.
- Always check the labels on cans or jars to determine how the contents should be stored. Many items besides fresh meats, vegetables, and dairy products need to be kept cold. For instance, mayonnaise and ketchup should go in the refrigerator after opening. If you've neglected to refrigerate items, it's usually best to throw them out.
- Some precautions will help make sure that foods that can be stored at room temperature remain safe. Potatoes and onions should not be stored under the sink because leakage from the pipes can damage the food. Potatoes don't belong in the refrigerator, either. Store them in a cool, dry place. Don't store foods near household cleaning products and chemicals.
- Check canned goods to see whether any are sticky on the outside. This may indicate a leak. Newly purchased cans that appear to be leaking should be returned to the store, which should notify the FDA.

Keep It Clean

- The first cardinal rule of safe food preparation in the home is: Keep everything clean.

The cleanliness rule applies to the areas where food is prepared and, most importantly, to the cook.
- Wash hands with warm water and soap for at least 20 seconds before starting to prepare a meal and after handling raw meat or poultry.
- Cover long hair with a net or scarf, and be sure that any open sores or cuts on the hands are completely covered. If the sore or cut is infected, stay out of the kitchen.
- Keep the work area clean and uncluttered. Wash countertops with a solution of 1 teaspoon of chlorine bleach to 1 quart of water or with a commercial kitchen cleaning agent diluted according to product directions. They're the most effective at getting rid of bacteria.
- Also, be sure to keep dishcloths clean because, when wet, they can harbor bacteria and may promote their growth. Wash dishcloths weekly in hot water in the washing machine.
- Sanitize the kitchen sink drain periodically by pouring down the sink a solution of 1 teaspoon of bleach to 1 quart of water or a commercial kitchen cleaning agent. Food particles get trapped in the drain and disposal and, along with the moistness, create an ideal environment for bacterial growth.
- Use smooth cutting boards made of hard maple or a non-porous material such as plastic and free of cracks and crevices. Avoid boards made of soft, porous materials. Wash cutting boards with hot water and soap, using a scrub brush. Then, sanitize them by washing in an automatic dishwasher or by rinsing with a solution of 1 teaspoon of chlorine bleach to 1 quart of water.
- Always wash and sanitize cutting boards after using them for raw foods, such as seafood or chicken, and before using them for ready-to-eat foods. Consider using one cutting board only for foods that will be cooked, such as raw fish, and another only for ready-to-eat foods, such as bread, fresh fruit, and cooked fish.
- Always use clean utensils and wash them between cutting different foods.
- Wash the lids of canned foods before opening to keep dirt from getting into the food. Also, clean the blade of the can opener after each use. Food processors and meat grinders should be taken apart and cleaned as soon as possible after they are used.
- Do not put cooked meat on an unwashed plate or platter that has held raw meat.
- Wash fresh fruits and vegetables thoroughly, rinsing under running water. Don't use soap or other detergents. If necessary—and appropriate—use a small scrub brush to remove surface dirt.

Keep Temperature Right

The second cardinal rule of safe home food preparation is: Keep hot foods hot and cold foods cold.

- Use a digital or dial food thermometer to ensure that meats are completely cooked. Insert the thermometer into the center of the food and

wait 30 seconds to ensure an accurate measurement. Beef, lamb, and veal should be cooked to at least 145°F (63°C); pork and ground beef to 160°F (71°C); whole poultry and thighs to 180°F (82°C); poultry breasts to 170°F (77°C); and ground chicken or turkey to 165°F (74°C).
- Eggs should be cooked until the white and the yolk are firm. Avoid foods containing raw eggs, such as homemade ice cream, mayonnaise, eggnog, cookie dough and cake batter, because they carry a *Salmonella* risk. Their commercial counterparts usually don't because they're made with pasteurized eggs. Cooking the egg-containing product to an internal temperature of at least 160°F (71°C) will kill the bacteria.
- Seafood should be thoroughly cooked to an internal temperature of at least 145°F (63°C). Fish that's ground or flaked, such as a fish cake, should be cooked to at least 155°F (68°C), and stuffed fish to at least 165°F (74°C).

If you don't have a food thermometer, look for other signs of doneness. For example:

- Fish is done when the thickest part becomes opaque and the fish flakes easily when poked with a fork.
- Shrimp can be simmered three to five minutes or until the shells turn red.
- Clams and mussels are steamed over boiling water until the shells open (five to 10 minutes). Then boil three to five minutes longer.
- Oysters should be sautéed, baked or boiled until plump, about five minutes.

Protect food from cross-contamination after cooking, and eat it promptly.

- Cooked foods should not be left standing on the table or kitchen counter for more than two hours. Disease-causing bacteria grow in temperatures between 40 and 140°F (4 and 60°C). Cooked foods that have been in this temperature range for more than two hours should not be eaten.
- If a dish is to be served hot, get it from the stove to the table as quickly as possible. Reheated foods should be brought to a temperature of at least 165°F (74°C). Keep cold foods in the refrigerator or on a bed of ice until serving. This rule is particularly important to remember in the summer months.
- After the meal, leftovers should be refrigerated as soon as possible. (Never mind that scintillating dinner table conversation!) Meats should be cut in slices of three inches or less and all foods should be stored in shallow containers to hasten cooling. Be sure to remove all the stuffing from roast turkey or chicken and store it separately. Giblets should also be stored separately. Leftovers should be used within three days.

And here are just a few more parting tips to keep your favorite dishes safe.

- Don't thaw meat and other frozen foods at room temperature. Instead, move them from the freezer to the refrigerator for a day or two; or defrost submerged in cold water. You can also defrost in the microwave

oven or during the cooking process. Cook foods immediately after defrosting in the microwave or cold water.
- Never taste any food that looks or smells "off" or comes out of leaking, bulging or severely damaged cans or jars with leaky lids.

Though all these dos and don'ts may seem overwhelming, remember, if you want to stay healthy, when it comes to food safety, the old saying "rules are made to be broken" does not apply!

VII. HACCP: A STATE-OF-THE-ART APPROACH TO FOOD SAFETY

The Food and Drug Administration Food Safety and Inspection Service (FSIS) adopted the Hazard Analysis and Critical Control Point Inspection Models Project to improve the nation's meat and poultry inspection system. The new system, known as HACCP, differs from the earlier system by focusing on potential problems and their early solution. This document, released in October 2001 by the FDA, lays out the rationale behind the program and the principals it adheres to, and details the timeline the government followed in initiating HACCP.

Space-age technology designed to keep food safe in outer space may soon become standard here on Earth.

The Food and Drug Administration has adopted a food safety program developed nearly 30 years ago for astronauts and is applying it to seafood and juice. The agency intends to eventually use it for much of the U.S. food supply. The program for the astronauts focuses on preventing hazards that could cause foodborne illnesses by applying science-based controls, from raw material to finished products. FDA's new system will do the same.

Traditionally, industry and regulators have depended on spot-checks of manufacturing conditions and random sampling of final products to ensure safe food. This approach, however, tends to be reactive, rather than preventive, and can be less efficient than the new system.

The new system is known as Hazard Analysis and Critical Control Point, or HACCP (pronounced hassip). Many of its principles already are in place in the FDA-regulated low-acid canned food industry. FDA also established HACCP for the seafood industry in a final rule [released] December 18, 1995, and for the juice industry in a final rule released January 19, 2001. The final rule for the juice industry will take effect on January 22, 2002, for large and medium businesses, January 21, 2003, for small businesses, and January 20, 2004, for very small businesses.

In 1998, the U.S. Department of Agriculture [...] established HACCP for meat and poultry processing plants, as well. Most of these establishments were required to start using HACCP by January 1999. Very small plants had until Jan. 25, 2000. (USDA regulates meat and poultry; FDA all other foods.)

FDA now is considering developing regulations that would establish HACCP as the food safety standard throughout other areas of the food industry, including both domestic and imported food products.

To help determine the degree to which such regulations would be feasible, the agency is conducting pilot HACCP programs with volunteer food companies. The programs have involved cheese, frozen dough, breakfast cereals, salad dressing, bread, flour and other products.

HACCP has been endorsed by the National Academy of Sciences, the Codex Alimentarius Commission (an international food standard–setting organization), and the National Advisory Committee on Microbiological Criteria for Foods.

A number of U.S. food companies already use the system in their manufacturing processes, and it is in use in other countries, including Canada.

What Is HACCP?

HACCP involves seven principles:

- *Analyze hazards.* Potential hazards associated with a food and measures to control those hazards are identified. The hazard could be biological, such as a microbe; chemical, such as a toxin; or physical, such as ground glass or metal fragments.
- *Identify critical control points.* These are points in a food's production—from its raw state through processing and shipping to consumption by the consumer—at which the potential hazard can be controlled or eliminated. Examples are cooking, cooling, packaging, and metal detection.
- *Establish preventive measures with critical limits for each control point.* For a cooked food, for example, this might include setting the minimum cooking temperature and time required to ensure the elimination of any harmful microbes.
- *Establish procedures to monitor the critical control points.* Such procedures might include determining how and by whom cooking time and temperature should be monitored.
- *Establish corrective actions to be taken when monitoring shows that a critical limit has not been met*—for example, reprocessing or disposing of food if the minimum cooking temperature is not met.
- *Establish procedures to verify that the system is working properly*—for example, testing time-and-temperature recording devices to verify that a cooking unit is working properly.
- *Establish effective recordkeeping to document the HACCP system.* This would include records of hazards and their control methods, the monitoring of safety requirements and action taken to correct potential problems. Each of these principles must be backed by sound scientific knowledge: for example, published microbiological studies on time and temperature factors for controlling foodborne pathogens.

Need for HACCP

New challenges to the U.S. food supply have prompted FDA to consider adopting a HACCP-based food safety system on a wider basis. One of the most important challenges is the increasing number of new food pathogens. For example, between 1973 and 1988, bacteria not previously recognized as important causes of food-borne illness—such as *Escherichia coli* O157:H7 and *Salmonella enteritidis*—became more widespread.

There also is increasing public health concern about chemical contamination of food: for example, the effects of lead in food on the nervous system.

Another important factor is that the size of the food industry and the diversity of products and processes have grown tremendously—in the amount of domestic food manufactured and the number and kinds of foods imported. At the same time, FDA and state and local agencies have the same limited level of resources to ensure food safety.

The need for HACCP in the United States, particularly in the seafood and juice industries, is further fueled by the growing trend in international trade for worldwide equivalence of food products and the Codex Alimentarious Commission's adoption of HACCP as the international standard for food safety.

Advantages

HACCP offers a number of advantages over the current system. Most importantly, HACCP:

- focuses on identifying [hazards] and preventing [them] from contaminating food
- is based on sound science
- permits more efficient and effective government oversight, primarily because the recordkeeping allows investigators to see how well a firm is complying with food safety laws over a period rather than how well it is doing on any given day
- places responsibility for ensuring food safety appropriately on the food manufacturer or distributor
- helps food companies compete more effectively in the world market
- reduces barriers to international trade.

VIII. NATIONAL SCHOOL LUNCH PROGRAM FACT SHEET

The National School Lunch Program (NSLP) was established under the National School Lunch Act in 1946, signed by President Harry Truman. The program is a federally assisted meal program that operates in public and nonprofit private schools and residential child care institutions. This July 2008 fact sheet provided by the USDA Food and Nutrition Service (FNS) details the specifics of the program requirements and related costs.

1. What Is the National School Lunch Program?

The National School Lunch Program is a federally assisted meal program operating in over 101,000 public and non-profit private schools and residential child care institutions. It provide[d] nutritionally balanced, low-cost or free lunches to more than 30.5 million children each school day in 2007. In 1998, Congress expanded the National School Lunch Program to include reimbursement for snacks served to children in afterschool educational and enrichment programs to include children through 18 years of age.

The Food and Nutrition Service administers the program at the Federal level. At the State level, the National School Lunch Program is usually administered by State education agencies, which operate the program through agreements with school food authorities.

2. How Does the National School Lunch Program Work?

Generally, public or nonprofit private schools of high school grade or under and public or nonprofit private residential child care institutions may participate in the school lunch program. School districts and independent schools that choose to take part in the lunch program get cash subsidies and donated commodities from the U.S. Department of Agriculture (USDA) for each meal they serve. In return, they must serve lunches that meet Federal requirements, and they must offer free or reduced price lunches to eligible children. School food authorities can also be reimbursed for snacks served to children through age 18 in afterschool educational or enrichment programs.

3. What Are the Nutritional Requirements for School Lunches?

School lunches must meet the applicable recommendations of the 1995 Dietary Guidelines for Americans, which recommend that no more than 30 percent of an individual's calories come from fat, and less than 10 percent from saturated fat. Regulations also establish a standard for school lunches to provide one-third of the Recommended Dietary Allowances of protein, Vitamin A, Vitamin C, iron, calcium, and calories.

School lunches must meet Federal nutrition requirements, but decisions about what specific foods to serve and how they are prepared are made by local school food authorities.

4. How Do Children Qualify for Free and Reduced-price Meals?

Any child at a participating school may purchase a meal through the National School Lunch Program. Children from families with incomes at or below 130 percent of the poverty level are eligible for free meals. Those with incomes between 130 percent and 185 percent of the poverty level are eligible for reduced-price meals, for which students can be charged no more than 40 cents. (For the period July 1, 2008, through June 30, 2009, 130 percent of the poverty level is $27,560 for a family of four; 185 percent is $39,220.)

Children from families with incomes over 185 percent of poverty pay a full price, though their meals are still subsidized to some extent. Local school food authorities set their own prices for full-price (paid) meals, but must operate their meal services as non-profit programs.

Table A.2 Lunch Reimbursement

Free lunches:	$2.57
Reduced-price lunches:	$2.17
Paid lunches:	$0.24
Free snacks:	$0.71
Reduced-price snacks:	$0.35
Paid snacks:	$0.06

[Courtesy of the USDA Food and Nutrition Service]

Afterschool snacks are provided to children on the same income eligibility basis as school meals. However, programs that operate in areas where at least 50 percent of students are eligible for free or reduced-price meals may serve all their snacks for free.

5. How Much Reimbursement Do Schools Get?

Most of the support USDA provides to schools in the National School Lunch Program comes in the form of a cash reimbursement for each meal served. The current (July 1, 2008 through June 30, 2009) basic cash reimbursement rates if school food authorities served less than 60% free and reduced price lunches during the second preceding school year are:

Higher reimbursement rates are in effect for Alaska and Hawaii, and for schools with high percentages of low-income students. For the latest reimbursement rates visit FNS website at http://www.fns.usda.gov/cnd/Governance/notices/naps/NAPs.htm.

6. What Other Support Do Schools Get from USDA?

In addition to cash reimbursements, schools are entitled by law to receive commodity foods, called "entitlement" foods, at a value of 20.75 cents for each meal served in Fiscal Year 2008–2009. Schools can also get "bonus" commodities as they are available from surplus agricultural stocks.

Through Team Nutrition USDA provides schools with technical training and assistance to help school food service staffs prepare healthful meals, and with nutrition education to help children understand the link between diet and health.

7. What Types of Foods Do Schools Get from USDA?

States select entitlement foods for their schools from a list of various foods purchased by USDA and offered through the school lunch program. Bonus foods are offered only as they become available through agricultural surplus. The variety of both entitlement and bonus commodities schools can get from USDA depends on quantities available and market prices.

A very successful project between USDA and the Department of Defense (DOD) has helped provide schools with fresh produce purchased through DOD. USDA has also worked with schools to help promote connections with local small farmers who may be able to provide fresh produce.

8. How Many Children Have Been Served Over the Years?

The National School Lunch Act in 1946 created the modern school lunch program, though USDA had provided funds and food to schools for many years prior to that. About 7.1 million children were participating in the National School Lunch Program by the end of its first year, 1946–47. By 1970, 22 million children were participating, and by 1980 the figure was nearly 27 million. In 1990, over 24 million children ate school lunch every day. In Fiscal Year 2007, more than 30.5 million children each day got their lunch through the National School Lunch Program. Since the modern program began, more than 187 billion lunches have been served.

9. How Much Does the Program Cost?

The National School Lunch Program cost $8.7 billion in [fiscal year] 2007. By comparison, the lunch program's total cost in 1947 was $70 million; in 1950, $119.7 million; in 1960, $225.8 million; in 1970, $565.5 million; in 1980, $3.2 billion; in 1990, $3.7 billion; and in 2000, $6.1 billion.

For More Information

For information on the operation of the National School Lunch Program and all the Child Nutrition Programs, contact the State agency in your state that is responsible for the administration of the programs. A listing of all our State agencies may be found on our web site at www.fns.usda.gov/cnd; select "Contact Us", then select "Child Nutrition Programs."

You may also contact us through the office of USDA, Food and Nutrition Service, Public Information Staff at 703-305-2286, or by mail at 3101 Park Center Drive, Room 914, Alexandria, Virginia 22302.

IX. SAMPLE MENUS FOR A 2000-CALORIE FOOD PATTERN

The USDA Food Guide Pyramid and related educational information offers consumers a graphic presentation of healthy food choices, as well as specific menu suggestions. The pyramid was initially released in 1992 with the objective of helping consumers better understand and apply the 1990 Dietary Guidelines. These sample menus represent the USDA recommended amounts of nutrients and food from each identified food group: grains, vegetables, fruits, milk, meat and beans, and oils.

Averaged over a week, this seven-day menu provides all of the recommended amounts of nutrients and food from each food group.

(Italicized foods are part of the dish or food that precedes [them].)

Table A.3 Sample Menus

Day 1	Day 2	Day 3	Day 4	Day 5	Day 6	Day 7
BREAKFAST	**BREAKFAST**	**BREAKFAST**	**BREAKFAST**	**BREAKFAST**	**BREAKFAST**	**BREAKFAST**
Breakfast burrito	Hot cereal	Cold cereal	1 whole wheat English muffin	Cold cereal	French toast	Pancakes
1 flour tortilla (7" diameter)	½ cup cooked oatmeal	1 cup bran flakes	2 tsp soft margarine	1 cup shredded wheat cereal	2 slices whole wheat French toast	3 buckwheat pancakes
1 scrambled egg (in 1 tsp soft margarine)	2 tbsp raisins	1 cup fat-free milk	1 tbsp jam or preserves	1 tbsp raisins	2 tsp soft margarine	2 tsp soft margarine
⅓ cup black beans*	1 tsp soft margarine	1 small banana	1 medium grapefruit	1 cup fat-free milk	2 tbsp maple syrup	3 tbsp maple syrup
2 tbsp salsa	½ cup fat-free milk	1 slice whole wheat toast	1 hard-cooked egg	1 small banana	½ medium grapefruit	½ cup strawberries
1 cup orange juice	1 cup orange juice	1 tsp soft margarine	1 unsweetened beverage	1 slice whole wheat toast	1 cup fat-free milk	¾ cup honeydew melon
1 cup fat-free milk		1 cup prune juice		1 tsp soft margarine		½ cup fat-free milk
				1 tsp jelly		
LUNCH	**LUNCH**	**LUNCH**	**LUNCH**	**LUNCH**	**LUNCH**	**LUNCH**
Roast beef sandwich	Taco salad	Tuna fish sandwich	White bean-vegetable soup	Smoked turkey sandwich	Vegetarian chili on baked potato	Manhattan clam chowder
1 whole grain sandwich bun	2 ounces tortilla chips	2 slices rye bread	1 ¼ cup vegetable soup	2 ounces whole wheat pita bread	1 cup kidney beans*	3 ounces canned clams (drained)
3 ounces lean roast beef	2 ounces ground turkey, sautéed in 2 tsp sunflower oil	3 ounces tuna (packed in water, drained)	½ cup white beans*	¼ cup romaine lettuce	½ cup tomato sauce	¾ cup mixed vegetables
2 slices tomato	½ cup black beans*	2 tsp mayonnaise	2 ounce breadstick	2 slices tomato	3 tbsp chopped onions	1 cup canned tomatoes*
¼ cup shredded lettuce	½ cup iceberg lettuce	1 tbsp diced celery	8 baby carrots	3 ounces sliced smoked turkey breast*	1 ounce lowfat cheese	10 whole wheat crackers*
⅛ cup sautéed mushrooms (in 1 tsp oil)	2 slices tomato	¼ cup shredded lettuce	1 cup fat-free milk	1 tbsp mayo-type salad dressing	1 tsp vegetable oil	1 medium orange
1 ½ ounce part-skim mozzarella cheese	1 ounce low-fat cheese	2 slices tomato		1 tsp yellow mustard	1 medium baked potato	1 cup fat-free milk
1 tsp yellow mustard	2 tbsp salsa	1 medium pear		½ cup apple slices	½ cup cantaloupe	
¾ cup baked potato wedges*	½ cup avocado	1 cup fat-free milk		1 cup tomato juice*	¾ cup lemonade	
1 tbsp ketchup	1 tsp lime juice					
1 unsweetened beverage	1 unsweetened beverage					

DINNER
Stuffed broiled salmon
5 ounce salmon filet
1 ounce bread stuffing mix
1 tbsp diced celery
2 tsp canola oil
1/2 cup saffron (white) rice
1 ounce slivered almonds
1/2 cup steamed broccoli
1 tsp soft margarine
1 cup fat-free milk

DINNER
Spinach lasagna
1 cup lasagna noodles, cooked (2 oz. dry)
2/3 cup cooked spinach
1/2 cup ricotta cheese
1/2 cup tomato sauce
1 ounce part-skim mozzarella cheese
1 ounce whole wheat roll
1 cup fat-free milk

DINNER
Roasted chicken breast
3 ounces boneless skinless chicken breast*
1 large baked sweet potato
1/2 cup peas and onions
1 tsp soft margarine
1 ounce whole wheat roll
1 tsp soft margarine
1 cup leafy greens salad
3 tsp sunflower oil and vinegar dressing

DINNER
Rigatoni with meat sauce
1 cup rigatoni pasta (2 oz. dry)
1/2 cup tomato sauce
2 ounces extra lean cooked ground beef (sautéed in 2 tsp vegetable oil)
3 tbsp grated Parmesan cheese
Spinach salad
1 cup baby spinach leaves
1/2 cup tangerine slices
1/2 ounce chopped walnuts
3 tsp sunflower oil and vinegar dressing
1 cup fat-free milk

DINNER
Grilled top loin steak
5 ounces grilled top loin steak
3/4 cup mashed potatoes
2 tsp soft margarine
1/2 cup steamed carrots
1 tbsp honey
2 ounces whole wheat dinner roll
1 tsp soft margarine
1 cup fat-free milk

DINNER
Hawaiian pizza
2 slices cheese pizza
1 ounce Canadian bacon
1/4 cup pineapple
2 tbsp mushrooms
2 tbsp chopped onions
Green salad
1 cup leafy greens
3 tsp sunflower oil and vinegar dressing
1 cup fat-free milk

DINNER
Vegetable stir-fry
4 ounces tofu (firm)
1/4 cup green and red bell peppers
1/2 cup bok choy
2 tbsp vegetable oil
1 cup brown rice
1 cup lemon-flavored iced tea

SNACKS
1 cup cantaloupe

SNACKS
1/2 oz dry-roasted almonds
1/4 cup pineapple
2 tbsp raisins

SNACKS
1/4 cup dried apricots
1 cup low-fat fruited yogurt

SNACKS
1 cup low-fat fruited yogurt

SNACKS
1 cup low-fat fruited yogurt

SNACKS
5 whole wheat crackers*
1/8 cup hummus
1/2 cup fruit cocktail (in water or juice)

SNACKS
1 ounce sunflower seeds*
1 large banana
1 cup low-fat fruited yogurt

* Starred items are foods that are labeled as no-salt-added, low-sodium, or low-salt versions of the foods. They can also be prepared from scratch with little or no added salt. All other foods are regular commercial products, which contain variable levels of sodium. Average sodium level of the 7-day menu assumes no salt added in cooking or at the table.

[Courtesy of USDA Center for Nutrition Policy and Promotion]

APPENDIX B

Nutrition Timeline

1747	British naval surgeon James Lind discovered a cure for scurvy.
1862	President Abraham Lincoln established the U.S. Department of Agriculture (USDA).
1883	Dr. Harvey W. Wiley was named chief chemist for the U.S. Bureau of Chemistry's food adulteration studies.
1888	W. O. Atwater was named the first director of the USDA Office of Experiment Stations.
1889	President Grover Cleveland elevated the USDA to a Cabinet-level department.
1894	Congress approved the first federal funding for nutrition research through a $10,000 agricultural appropriations bill.
1896	W. O. Atwater and A. P. Bryant published *The Chemical Composition of American Food Materials,* known as *Bulletin No. 28.*
1897	Dutch physician Christian Eijkman discovered a cure for beriberi.
1902	Dr. Harvey W. Wiley recruited young men as human guinea pigs to test food additives.
1903	French physicist Antoine H. Becquerel discovered radioactivity, and shared the year's Nobel Prize in physics with Marie and Pierre Curie.
1904	American biologist Samuel Prescott linked radiation with food safety.
1906	Upton Sinclair's novel *The Jungle* added to U.S. food safety fears.
1906	The Pure Food and Drug Act was passed by Congress and signed by President Theodore Roosevelt, prohibiting food adulteration and misbranding.
1906	The Meat Inspection Act was passed by Congress.
1916	The USDA printed its first food guide, *Food for Young Children.*
1921	A U.S. patent was granted for the use of X-ray technology to kill bacteria in pork.

NUTRITION TIMELINE

1925 The first home mechanical refrigerator, Frigidaire, was sold.

1927 The Bureau of Chemistry was reorganized into the Food, Drug and Insecticide Administration and the Bureau of Chemistry and Soils.

1930 The Food, Drug and Insecticide Administration was renamed the Food and Drug Administration (FDA).

1933 The FDA recommended revision of the 1906 Pure Food and Drug Act.

1937 The medicine Elixir Sulfanilamide killed over 100 people, and dramatized the need for improved U.S. drug safety laws.

1937 The McDonald brothers opened the first drive-in restaurant.

1938 The Federal Food, Drug and Cosmetic (FDC) Act was passed by Congress.

1938 Flemmie Pansy Kittrell became the first African American woman to receive a PhD in nutrition, earning her degree with honors.

1940 Walter G. Campbell was appointed the first Commissioner of Food and Drugs for the FDA.

1941 The Recommended Dietary Allowances (RDAs) were published.

1946 The National School Lunch Act was passed by Congress.

1949 The FDA published industry guidelines, "Procedures for the Appraisal of the Toxicity of Chemicals in Food."

1950 The Delaney Committee called for a congressional investigation into food additive safety.

1953 President Dwight Eisenhower addressed the United Nations General Assembly on "Atoms for Peace."

1954 The Miller Pesticide Amendment established safety limits for pesticide residues on raw agricultural commodities.

1956 The USDA published the "Basic Four" food guide.

1958 The Delaney Clause was added to the Pure Food and Drug Act, banning food additives shown to cause cancer in laboratory animals.

1958 The FDA released the first "generally recognized as safe" (GRAS) list of substances, recognizing almost 200 substances.

1959 A recall of the U.S. cranberry crop three weeks before Thanksgiving prompted the first and only FDA-generated safety label.

1960 The Color Additive Amendment was enacted.

1963 The FDA approved irradiation of wheat, flour, and canned bacon.

1965 The USDA required labels on irradiated foods.

1966 The Child Nutrition Act began the school breakfast program.

1968 The FDA rejected radiation-sterilized ham for safety reasons.

1969 President Richard Nixon held the White House Conference on Food, Nutrition and Health, and ordered FDA review of the GRAS list.

1971 Frances Moore Lappé published *Diet for a Small Planet*.

NUTRITION TIMELINE

1973	Voluntary nutrition labeling appeared on food packages.
1976	The Vitamins and Minerals Amendments, or Proxmire Amendments, blocked FDA efforts to regulate vitamins and supplements.
1977	A U.S. Senate Committee released *Dietary Goals for the United States*.
1979	The FDA established the Bureau of Foods Irradiated Food Committee (BFIFC).
1980	The USDA and the Department of Health and Human Services (HHS) released the official *Dietary Guidelines for Americans*.
1980	The USDA inherited the U.S. Army irradiation program.
1982	Scientists first transferred genes between plant species.
1984	The USDA released the Food Guide Pyramid in cooperation with the American National Red Cross.
1985	The FDA approved irradiation of pork to control trichinosis.
1985	The first genetically modified (GM) crop trials began around the world.
1986	The FDA approved irradiation for a number of fruits, vegetables, and grains.
1986	The Reagan administration divided food safety responsibilities between three federal agencies.
1989	The FDA issued a nationwide recall of L-tryptophan supplements, and banned imports of L-tryptophan, after 38 people died.
1990	Congress passed the Nutrition Labeling and Education Act, making nutrition labeling mandatory.
1990	Congress passed the Organic Foods Production Act (OFPA), giving farmers an official organic standard.
1990	The FDA approved irradiation of poultry.
1992	The FDA and Food Safety and Inspection Service of the USDA released new easy-to-follow food labels.
1992	The USDA and HHS released the "Food Guide Pyramid."
1992	The British epidemic of bovine spongiform encephalopathy (BSE), or "mad cow disease," reached its peak of 37,000 cases per year.
1994	Congress approved the Dietary Supplement Health and Education Act.
1994	The first GM food, the Flavr Savr tomato, was approved for sale in the U.S.
1995	The World Trade Organization (WTO) was created to oversee international free trade benefits.
1997	The Center for Food Safety, a food activism group, was established.
1997	The FDA approved irradiation of red meat.
1998	A small group of scientists, environmentalists, consumer advocates, and religious leaders sued the FDA over GM food policies.
1998	England's Prince Charles criticized British scientists for playing God through research into genetically modified organisms.

1998	Researcher Arpad Pusztai claimed on British television that GM potatoes harmed rats.
1998	The U.S. government initiated plans to consolidate FDA laboratories nationwide, from 19 facilities to 9 by 2014.
2000	StarLink corn was detected in Taco Bell taco shells. Kraft Foods, Inc., issued an immediate recall.
2000	FDA regulations were changed to allow irradiation of fresh eggs to control salmonella.
2002	Maine farmer Arthur Harvey filed a civil lawsuit against Secretary of Agriculture Ann Veneman, to challenge the National Organic Program (NOP).
2003	The National Academy of Sciences released a report supporting Hazard Analysis and Critical Control Point (HACCP) food safety practices.
2004	Genetically modified corn was approved for planting in Britain.
2004	The FDA banned supplements containing ephedrine alkaloids, due to a risk of serious health problems.
2005	The USDA released an updated *Dietary Guidelines for Americans*.
2005	The U.S. Court of Appeals ruled in favor of Arthur Harvey on key issues in the Harvey organics lawsuit.
2006	Trans fat content became required on nutrition labels.
2006	Production of Flavr Savr genetically engineered tomatoes was halted.
2006	RDAs were renamed Reference Daily Intakes (RDIs).
2007	The National Climate March in London was held to focus on the link between climate change and the environmental effects of livestock farming and animal agriculture.
2008	French President Nicolas Sarkozy banned strains of GM corn in France.
2008	The State of California passed legislation mandating calorie counts on chain restaurant menus and menu boards.
2008	The City of Los Angeles passed a fast-food moratorium to stop any new fast food or freestanding quick-service restaurants from opening within a 32-square-mile area in the southern part of the city.

Appendix C

Directory of Organizations

American Council on Science and Health (ACSH)
Address: 1995 Broadway, Second Floor, New York, NY 10023-5860
Web address: **www.acsh.org**

American Diabetes Association (ADA)
Address: 1701 North Beauregard Street, Alexandria, VA 22311
Web address: **www.diabetes.org**

American Dietetic Association (ADA)
Address: 120 South Riverside Plaza, Suite 2000, Chicago, IL 60606-6995
Web address: **www.eatright.org**

American Heart Association (AHA)
Address: 7272 Greenville Avenue, Dallas, TX 75231
Web address: **www.americanheart.org**

Centers for Disease Control and Prevention (CDC)
Address: 1600 Clifton Road, NE, Atlanta, GA 30333
Web address: **www.cdc.gov**

Center for Food Safety
Address: 666 Pennsylvania Avenue, SE, Suite 302, Washington, DC 20003
Web address: **www.centerforfoodsafety.org**

Center for Foodborne Illness Research and Prevention (CFI)
Address: P.O. Box 206, Grove City, PA 16127
Web address: **www.foodborneillness.org**

Center for Science in the Public Interest (CSPI)
Address: 1875 Connecticut Avenue, NW, Suite 300, Washington, DC 20009
Web address: **www.cspinet.org**

Consumers Union
Address: 101 Truman Avenue, Yonkers, NY 10703-1057
Web address: **www.consumersunion.org**

Council for Responsible Nutrition (CRN)
Address: 1828 L Street, NW, Suite 510, Washington DC 20036-5114
Web address: **www.crnusa.org**

EarthSave International
Address: PO Box 96, New York, NY 10108
Web address: **www.earthsave.org**

Food and Drug Administration (FDA)/U.S. Department of Health and Human Services
Address: 200 Independence Avenue, SW, Washington, DC 20201
Web address: **www.fda.gov**

Food and Nutrition Information Center (FNIC)/U.S. Department of Agriculture
Address: 10301 Baltimore Avenue, Room 105, Beltsville, MD 20705-2351
Web address: **www.nal.usda.gov/fnic**

Food and Water Watch
Address: 1616 P Street, NW, Suite 300, Washington, DC 20036
Web address: **www.foodandwaterwatch.org**

Food First
Address: 398 60th Street, Oakland, CA 94618
Web address: **www.foodfirst.org**

Friends of the Earth
Address: 1717 Massachusetts Avenue, NW, Suite 600, Washington, DC 20036
Web address: **www.foe.org**

Fruits and Veggies Matter
Address: Centers for Disease Control and Prevention, 4770 Buford Highway, NE, MS/K-24, Atlanta, GA 30341-3717
Web address: **www.fruitsandveggiesmatter.gov**

Greenpeace
Address: 702 H Street, NW, Suite 300, Washington, DC 20001
Web address: **www.greenpeace.org**

DIRECTORY OF ORGANIZATIONS

Healthfinder/U.S. Department of Health and Human Services
Address: 200 Independence Avenue, SW, Washington, DC 20201
Web address: **www.healthfinder.gov**

Institute for Agriculture and Trade Policy (IATP)
Address: 2105 First Avenue South, Minneapolis, MN 55404
Web address: **www.iatp.org**

International Food Information Council (IFIC)
Address: 1100 Connecticut Avenue, NW, Suite 430, Washington, DC 20036
Web address: **www.ific.org**

International Society for Orthomolecular Medicine (ISOM)
Address: 16 Florence Avenue, Toronto, Ontario, Canada M2N 1E9
Web address: **www.orthomed.org**

Monsanto
Address: 800 North Lindberg Boulevard, St. Louis, MO 63167
Web address: **www.monsanto.com**

MyPyramid/U.S. Department of Agriculture
Address: USDA Center for Nutrition Policy and Promotion 3101 Park Center Drive, Room 1034, Alexandria, VA 22302-1594.
Web address: **www.mypyramid.gov**

National Academy of Sciences (NAS) Institute of Medicine/Food Nutrition Board
Address: 500 Fifth Street, NW, Washington, DC 20001
Web address: **www.iom.edu**

National Cancer Institute (NCI)
Address: 9000 Rockville Pike, Building 31, Room 10A19, Bethesda, MD 20892-2582
Web address: **www.nci.nih.gov**

National Center for Food and Agriculture Policy (NCFAP)
Address: 1616 P Street, NW, First Floor, Washington, DC 20036
Web address: **www.ncfap.org**

Nutrition.gov/U.S. Department of Agriculture
Address: 10301 Baltimore Avenue, Beltsville, MD 20705-2351
Web address: **www.nutrition.gov**

Organic Consumers Association (OCA)
Address: 6771 South Silver Hill Drive, Finland, MN 55603
Web address: **www.organicconsumers.org**

People for the Ethical Treatment of Animals (PETA)
Address: 501 Front Street, Norfolk, VA 23510
Web address: **www.peta.org**

President's Council on Food Safety
Address: 200 Independence Avenue, SW, Washington, DC 20201
Web address: **www.foodsafety.gov**

Rodale Institute
Address: 611 Siegfriedale Road, Kutztown, PA 19530-9320
Web address: **www.rodaleinstitute.org**

Safe Tables Our Priority (STOP)
Address: 3149 Dundee Road, #276, Northbrook, IL 60062
Web address: **www.safetables.org**

Union of Concerned Scientists
Address: 2 Brattle Square, Cambridge, MA 02238-9105
Web address: **www.ucsusa.org**

U.S. Environmental Protection Agency (EPA)
Address: 1200 Pennsylvania Avenue, NW, Washington, DC 20460
Web address: **www.epa.gov**

Vegetarian Resource Group (VRG)
Address: P.O. Box 1463, Baltimore, MD 21203
Web address: **www.vrg.org**

World Health Organization (WHO)
Address: 525 23rd street, NW, Washington, DC 20037
Web address: **www.who.int/en**

World Trade Organization (WTO)
Address: Rue de Lausanne 154, Ch-1211 Geneva 21, Switzerland
Web address: **www.wto.org**

NOTES

CHAPTER 1

1. Barbara Kingsolver, Steven L. Hopp, and Camille Kingsolver, *Animal, Vegetable, Miracle: A Year of Food Life* (New York: HarperCollins, 2007), 5.
2. "Johannes Baptista van Helmont," in *Biography Resource Center* (Farmington Hills, MI: Gale, 2008), http://galenet.galegroup.com/Servlet/BioRC..
3. "Frederick Gowland Hopkins," in *Biography Resource Center* (Farmington Hills, MI: Gale, 2008), http://galenet.galegroup.com/Servlet/BioRC.
4. "The Next War," in *American Decades Primary Sources*, vol. 2, *1910–1919*, ed. Cynthia Rose (Detroit: Gale, 2004), 466.
5. Dan Hurley, *Natural Causes: Death, Lies, and Politics in America's Vitamin and Herbal Supplement Industry* (New York: Broadway Books, 2006), 38.
6. Ibid., 42.

CHAPTER 2

1. Season Solorio, "More Consumers Consider Themselves 'Regular' Supplement Users, Annual Survey Results Show," Council for Responsible Nutrition, http://www.crnusa.org/prpdfs/CRN_PR_100407_ConsumerConfidence.pdf.

CHAPTER 3

1. Marc T. Law, *History of Food and Drug Regulation in the United States*, in *EH.Net Encyclopedia*, ed. Robert Whaples (EH.Net, 2004), http://eh.net/encyclopedia/article/Law.Food.and.Drug.Regulation.
2. U.S. Food and Drug Administration, "FDA's Mission Statement," "Protecting Consumers, Promoting Public Health," http://www.fda.gov/opacom/morechoices/mission.html.http://www.fda.gov/oc/opacom/fda101/fda101text.html

CHAPTER 4

1. Centers for Disease Control and Prevention Food Safety Office, updated January 19, 2009, http://www.cdc.gov/foodsafety/.
2. Myrna Chandler Goldstein and Mark A. Goldstein, *Controversies in Food and Nutrition* (Westport, CT: Greenwood Press, 2002), 29.
3. Ibid., 30.
4. "Irradiation in the Production, Processing and Handling of Food," *Federal Register* 51, no. 75 (April 18, 1986): 13376 (Food and Drug Administration; Department of Health and Human Services).
5. George H. Pauli and Clyde A. Takeguchi, "Irradiation of Foods: An FDA Perspective," *Food Reviews International* 2, no. 1 (1986): 90, www.cfsan.fad.gov/~acrobat/irrahist.pdf.
6. Ibid., 92.
7. Ibid., 93.
8. "Food Additives Intended for Use in Processing of Canned Bacon: Proposed Revocations," *Federal Register* 33, no. 166 (August 24, 1968): 12055 (Food and Drug Administration).
9. Pauli and Takeguchi, "Irradiation of Foods: An FDA Perspective," 95.
10. "Policy for Irradiated Foods: Advance Notice of Proposed Procedures for the Regulation of Irradiated Foods for Human Consumption," *Federal Register* 46, no. 59 (March 27, 1981): 18992 (Food and Drug Administration).
11. "Irradiation . . .," *Federal Register* 51, no. 75 (April 18, 1986): 13382.
12. Food and Water Watch, "Irradiation: Expensive, Ineffective, and Impractical," http://www.foodandwaterwatch.org/food/foodirradiation/irradiation-facts.
13. "Position of the American Dietetic Association: Food Irradiation," *Journal of the American Dietetic Association* 100, no. 2 (February 2000): 246–253.
14. Ahmed El Amin, "Irradiation Regulation Remains Inconsistent Worldwide," *Food Navigator.com*, February 15, 2006, http://www.foodnavigator.com/news/printNewsBis.asp?id=65836.
15. World Health Organization, "High-Dose Irradiation: Wholesomeness of Food Irradiated with Doses above 10 kGy" (report of a joint FAO/IAEA/WHO study group, Geneva, September 15–20, 1997), Technical Report Series, no. 890: 161, http://www.who.int/foodsafety/publications/fs_management/irradiation/en/.

CHAPTER 5

1. Margaret Mellon and Jane Rissler, "Environmental Effects of Genetically Modified Food Crops: Recent Experiences" (paper presented at "Genetically Modified Foods—the American Experience," Copenhagen, June 12–13, 2003), reproduced by

Union of Concerned Scientists, http://www.ucusa.org/ food_and_agriculture/science_and_impacts/impacts_genetic_engineering/environmental-effects-of.html: 5.
2. John E. Losey, Linda S. Rayor, and Maureen E. Carter, "Transgenic Pollen Harms Monarch Larvae," *Nature* 399, no. 6733 (May 20, 1999): 214.
3. James Kanter, "EU Officials Propose Ban on Genetically Modified Corn Seeds," *International Herald Tribune,* November 21, 2007.
4. Jennifer A. Thomson, *Seeds for the Future* (Ithaca, NY: Cornell University Press, 2007), xviii.
5. Geoffrey S. Becker and Tadlock Cowan, "Agricultural Biotechnology: Background and Recent Issues," *Congressional Research Service (CRS) Reports and Issue Briefs,* September 2006: 4.
6. Center for Food Safety, "Genetically Engineered Food," http://www.centerforfoodsafety. org/geneticall7.cfm.
7. Steven M. Druker, "A Report on the Results of *Alliance for Bio-Integrity v. Shalala,* et al.," Alliance for Bio-Integrity, October 1, 2003, http://www.biointegrity.org/report-on-lawsuit.htm.
8. Andy Rees, *Genetically Modified Food: A Short Guide for the Confused* (Ann Arbor, MI: Pluto Press, 2006), 13.
9. Ian Sample, "The Return Of GM: Biotech Firm Mans Barricades as Campaigners Vow to Stop Trials: Small Field Near Cambridge the Latest Battleground in Fight to Prevent GM Trials," *Guardian,* February 16, 2008: 6.
10. Ibid.
11. Kathleen Hart, Eating in the Dark: America's Experiment with Genetically Engineered Food (New York: Pantheon Books, 2002), 119.
12. Ibid., 49.
13. Ibid., 25.
14. Rees, *Genetically Modified Food,* 7.
15. K. Lee Lerner and Brenda Wilmoth Lerner, eds., *Biotechnology: Changing Life through Science* (Farmington Hills, MI: Thomson Gale, 2007), 385.
16. Jason Simpkins and William Patalon III, "Monsanto Reaps Huge Rewards from Its Blossoming Seed Business," *MoneyMorning.com,* January 7, 2008. http:// www.moneymorning.com/2008/01/07/monsanto-reaps-huge-rewards-from-its-blossoming-seed-business/.

CHAPTER 6

1. Michael F. Jacobson, "Supplement Scams," *Nutrition Action Healthletter,* September 2007: 2.
2. Dan Hurley, *Natural Causes: Death, Lies, and Politics in America's Vitamin and Herbal Supplement Industry* (New York: Broadway Books, 2006), 166.

3. Season Solorio, "More Consumers Consider Themselves Regular Supplement Users, Annual Survey Results Show," *Council for Responsible Nutrition,* October 4, 2007, http://www.crnusa.org/prpdfs/CRN_PR_100407_ConsumerConfidence.pdf.
4. E. Ernst, V. S. Vassiliou, J. P. Pelletier, D. O. Clegg, and D. J. Reda, "Glucosamine and Chondroitin Sulfate for Knee Osteoarthritis," *New England Journal of Medicine* 354, no. 20 (May 18, 2006): 2184–2185.
5. "Toxic Herb Sold via Internet," *Better Nutrition* 66, no. 1 (January 2004): 22.
6. Thomas P. Cheung, Charlie Xue, Kelvin Leung, Kelvin Chan, and Chun G. Li, "Aristolochic Acids Detected in Some Raw Chinese Medicinal Herbs and Manufactured Herbal Products," *Clinical Toxicology* 44, no. 4 (June 2006): 371.
7. Gardiner Harris, "For FDA, a Major Backlog Overseas," *Virginian-Pilot*, January 29, 2008: 10.
8. Andrew W. Saul, "Vitamin Safety," *DoctorYourself.com,* http://www.doctoryourself.com/safety.html.
9. National Health Federation, "The NHF Declaration of Health-Freedom Rights," http://www.thenhf.com/declaration.htm.
10. Bonnie Liebman, "Confusion at the Vitamin Counter: Too Little or Too Much?" *Nutrition Action Healthletter,* November 2007: 3.
11. Ibid.
12. Ibid., 4.

CHAPTER 7

1. Marianne Lavelle and Kent Graber, "Fixing the Food Crisis," *U.S. News and World Report,* May 19, 2008: 42.
2. Neal Barnard, "Meat's Striking Out," *USA Today,* May 21, 2008, sec. A: 11.
3. American Dietetic Association, "Position of the American Dietetic Association and Dietitians of Canada: Vegetarian Diets," *Journal of the American Dietetic Association* 103, no. 6 (June 2003): 748–765.
4. Charles Stahler. "How Many Adults Are Vegetarian?" *Vegetarian Journal*, no. 4 (2006), www.vrg.org/journal/vj2006issue4/vj2006issue4poll.htm.
5. Frances Moore Lappé, *Diet for a Small Planet* (New York: Random House, 1982), 8.
6. Lavelle and Graber, 42.
7. American Institute for Cancer Research, "Recommendations for Cancer Prevention," *AICR Diet and Health Guidelines for Cancer Prevention*, http://www.aicr.org/site/-Page Server?pagename=dc_home_guides.
8. Jennifer Horsman and Jamie Flowers, *Please Don't Eat the Animals: All the Reasons You Need to Be a Vegetarian* (Sanger, CA: Wood Dancer Press, 2007), 37.
9. American Cancer Society, "Cancer Prevention and Early Detection: Facts and Figures, 2007" (Atlanta, GA: American Cancer Society, 2007), http://www.cancer.org/docroot/STT/content/STT_1x_Cancer_Prevention_and_Early_Detection_Facts__Figures_2007.asp.

10. Horsman, *Please Don't Eat the Animals,* 37.
11. Ibid., 8.
12. Peter Singer and Jim Mason, *The Ethics of What We Eat: Why Our Food Choices Matter* (Emmaus, PA: Rodale, 2006), 6.
13. Ibid., 23.
14. Ibid., 24.
15. Ibid., 43.
16. David Wallinga, "Playing Chicken: Avoiding Arsenic in Your Meat" (Minneapolis, MN: Institute for Agriculture and Trade Policy, 2006), 5.
17. Ibid., 6.
18. Ibid., 11.
19. Ibid., 8.
20. Ibid., 5.
21. Lance B. Price, Elizabeth Johnson, Rocio Vailes, and Ellen Silbergeld, "Fluoroquinolone-Resistant Campylobacter Isolates from Conventional and Antibiotic-Free Chicken Products," *Environmental Health Perspectives* 113, no. 5 (May 2005): 557.
22. "Dirty Birds: Even Premium Chickens Harbor Dangerous Bacteria," *Consumer Reports*, January 2007: 20.
23. Colin Spencer, *The Heretic's Feast: A History of Vegetarianism* (London: University Press of New England, 1995), 328.

CHAPTER 8

1. "National Organic Program: Proposed Amendment to the National List of Allowed and Prohibited Substances," *Federal Register* 73, no. 135 (July 14, 2008): 40200.
2. Patrick Holden, "Howard's Way," *The Ecologist* 31, no. 5 (June 2001): 30.
3. Ibid., 30.
4. Ward Greene, "Guru of the Organic Food Cult," *New York Times Magazine,* June 6, 1971: 57.
5. Ibid., 55.
6. Cathy Greene, "Organic Labeling," In *Economics of Food Labeling,* Elise Golan et al., Agricultural Economic Report no. 793 (USDA Economic Research Service, January 2001), http://www.ers.usda.gov/publications/aer793/aer793g.pdf.
7. Samuel Fromartz, *Organic, Inc.: Natural Foods and How They Grew* (Orlando, FL: Harcourt, 2006), 109.
8. Michael Pollan, *The Omnivore's Dilemma: A Natural History of Four Meals* (New York: Penguin Press, 2006), 164.
9. Kathryn Schuett, "Organic Valley: Celebrating 20 Years of Doing Good and Doing Well," *Organic Processing Magazine*, May–June 2008, http://www.organicprocessing.com/magazine.htm.
10. Barbara Kingsolver, Steven L. Hopp, and Camille Kingsolver, *Animal, Vegetable, Miracle: A Year of Food Life* (New York: HarperCollins, 2007), 206.

11. Myrna Chandler Goldstein and Mark A. Goldstein, *Controversies in Food and Nutrition* (Westport, CT: Greenwood Press, 2002), 196.
12. David Schardt, "Organic Food: Worth the Price?" *Nutrition Action Healthletter,* July–August 2007: 3.
13. Phillippe Grandjean et al., "The Faroes Statement: Human Health Effects of Developmental Exposure to Chemicals in Our Environment," *Basic and Clinical Pharmacology and Toxicology* 102, no. 2 (February 2008): 74.
14. Craig Minowa, "U.S. Government Facts: Children's Chemical and Pesticide Exposure via Food Products" (Organic Consumers Association, July 2005), http://www.organicconsumers.org/organic/wic-faq.pdf.
15. Ibid.
16. Kingsolver et al., *Animal, Vegetable, Miracle,* 165.
17. Charles Benbrook, Xin Zhao, Jaime Yanez, Neal Davies, and Preston Andrews, "New Evidence Confirms the Nutritional Superiority of Plant-Based Organic Foods," *Organic Center Critical Issue Report,* March 2008: 42
18. Felicity Lawrence, "Organic Milk Higher in Nutrients," *Guardian*, January 7, 2005: 10.
19. Benbrook et al., "New Evidence Confirms . . .," 42.
20. Joshua L. Posner, Jon O. Baldock, and Janet L. Hedtcke, "Organic and Conventional Production Ssystems in the Wisconsin Integrated Cropping Systems Trials: I. Productivity 1990–2002," *Agronomy Journal* 100 (2008): 253.
21. Paul Mäder et al., "Soil Fertility and Biodiversity in Organic Farming," *Science* 296, no. 5573 (May 31, 2002): 1694.
22. Fromartz, *Organic, Inc.,* 247.

CHAPTER 9

1. "*E. coli* Outbreak: Questions Loom on Food Safety," *Tulsa World,* September 4, 2008, sec. A: 14.
2. Eskin, Sandra B., Nancy Donley, Donna Rosenbaum, and Karen Taylor Mitchell. "Ten Years After the Jack-in-the-Box Outbreak Why Are People Still Dying from Contaminated Food?" 2003:9. http://www.safetables.org/communications/special_events_reports.cfm.
3. Ibid.
4. U.S. Department of Agriculture Economic Research Service, "Food Illness Cost Calculator: *Salmonella*," http://www.ers.usda.gov/data/foodborneillness/salm_Intro.asp.
5. Serrano, Alfonso, "How Safe is Imported Food?" *CBSnews.com,* April 16, 2007.
6. Upton Sinclair, *The Jungle* (New York: Buccaneer Books, 1984), 67.
7. U.S. Department of Agriculture Food Safety and Inspection Service, "Celebrating 100 Years of the Federal Meat Inspection Act (FMIA)" (May 15, 2006), http://www.fsis.usda.gov/About_FSIS/100_Years_FMIA/index.asp.
8. Marion Nestle, *What to Eat* (New York: North Point Press, 2006), 266.

9. T. R. Callaway, T. S. Edrington, R. C. Anderson, J. A. Byrd, and D. J. Nisbet, "Gastrointestinal Microbial Ecology and the Safety of Our Food Supply as Related to *Salmonella*," *Journal of Animal Science* 86, no. 14 (April 2008):E163-E172.
10. Lisa Sylvester, interview by Lou Dobbs, *Lou Dobbs Tonight*, CNN, June 20, 2008.
11. Julie Schmit, "U.S. Food Imports Outrun FDA Resources," *USA Today*, March 19, 2007, sec. B: 1.
12. Andrew Martin and Griff Palmer, "China Not Sole Source of Dubious Food," *New York Times*, July 12, 2007, sec. C: 1.
13. Lauran Neergaard, "The COOL Law: Country-of-Origin Labeling of Foods," *Virginian-Pilot*, September 30, 2008: 3.
14. Annys Shin, "Does Ethanol Raise Risks?" *Washington Post*, November 4, 2008, sec. H: 1.
15. Scott Hume, "Bush Boosts Food-Safety Budgets: Impact of Mad Cow Disease Incident Is Clear in Research and Testing Funds," *Restaurants and Institutions*, March 15, 2004: 60.
16. Jennifer Barone, "Milk Drinkers More Likely to Have Twins," *Discover* 28, no. 1 (January 2007): 48.
17. Nicholas Bakalar, "Rise in Rate of Twin Births May Be Tied to Dairy Case," *New York Times*, May 30, 2006, http://www.nytimes.com/2006/05/30/health/30twin.html.
18. "Overview." U.S. Food and Drug Administration Center for Food Safety and Applied Nutrition, February 2001. http://www.cfsan.fad.gov/~lrd/cfsan4.html.

CHAPTER 10

1. Eric Schlosser and Charles Wilson, *Chew on This: Everything You Don't Want to Know about Fast Food* (Houghton Mifflin: Boston, 2006), 10.
2. Paul Roberts, *The End of Food* (Houghton Mifflin: Boston, 2008), 99.
3. Corby Kummer, "Fat City," *Atlantic Monthly* 299, no. 2 (March 2007): 121.
4. Anne Kingston and Nicholas Kohler, "L.A.'S Fast-Food Drive-By: A City Council's Ban on Fast-Food Chains Is a Provocative Social Experiment," *Maclean's* 121, no. 33 (August 25, 2008): 36.
5. Ibid., 36.
6. Ibid, 37.
7. Michael Pollan, *The Omnivore's Dilemma* (Penguin Books: New York. 2006), 102.
8. U.S. Department of Health and Human Services Centers for Disease Control and Prevention, "Physical Activity and Good Nutrition: Essential Elements to Prevent Chronic Diseases and Obesity 2008" (February 2008), 2, http://www.cdc.gov/nccdphp/ publications/aag/pdf/dnpa.pdf.
9. Pam Belluck, "Obese Kids Show Early Signs of Heart Disease," *Virginian Pilot,* November 12, 2008: 4.
10. Annie Bell Muzaurieta. "Are School Lunches Causing Childhood Obesity?" *The DailyGreen.com,* November 3, 2008.

11. Physicians Committee for Responsible Medicine, "Healthy School Lunches: National School Lunch Program Background," http://www.healthyschoollunches.org/background/ nutrition.html.
12. Schlosser and Wilson, *Chew on This,* 56.
13. Amanda Spake and Mary Brophy Marcus, "A Fat Nation," *U.S. News and World Report,* August 19, 2002: 40.
14. Ibid., 40.
15. Schlosser and Wilson, *Chew on This,* 7.
16. Bonnie Liebman, "The Changing American Diet: A Report Card," *Nutrition Action Healthletter* 29, no. 10 (December 2002): 8.
17. Thomas H. Maugh, "Link Found between Drinking Soda, Even Diet, and Disease," *Virginian-Pilot,* July 7, 2007: 5.
18. Dan Collins, "McDonald's Wins Fat Fight," *CBSnews.com,* January 22, 2003, http://www.cbsnews.com/stories/2003/01/22/health/main537520.shtml.

Glossary

amino acids: Organic compounds composed of carbon, hydrogen, oxygen, nitrogen, and in some cases sulfur, bonded in formations. There are eight amino acids that cannot be manufactured by the body and must be obtained from the diet.

bacteria: The plural for bacterium, a single-cell microorganism without nuclei. Some bacteria are infectious.

beriberi: A disease caused by a deficiency of thiamine and characterized by nerve and gastrointestinal disorders.

biotoxin: Any poison made by a living organism.

bovine spongiform encephalopathy (BSE): A progressive neurological disorder of cattle that results from infection by an unusual transmissible agent called a prion. There is evidence that Creutzfeldt-Jakob disease (CJD) is caused by eating beef from BSE-infected cattle.

Campylobacter jejuni: One of the most common causes of diarrhea illness in the United States. It can lead to arthritis, or, in rare cases, can develop into a disease called Guillain-Barré syndrome. Most cases of campylobacteriosis are associated with eating raw or undercooked poultry or meat, or with cross-contamination of other foods by these items.

carbohydrate: A compound consisting of carbon, hydrogen, and oxygen, found in plants and used as a food by humans and other animals.

cells: Tiny units of which living things are made.

cholera: An illness caused by bacteria, spread by consuming contaminated food or water. Once a huge public health problem, the disease has been virtually eliminated in the developed world.

Clostridium botulinum: This bacterium lives in the soil and is sometimes found in low-acid foods. It produces a toxin that causes botulism, a disease characterized by muscle paralysis.

complete protein: A protein that includes all eight essential amino acids.

contamination: The unintended presence of harmful substances or microorganisms in food.

Creutzfeldt-Jakob disease (CJD) & vCJD: CJD is a human neurodegenerative disorder caused by prions, with an unusually long incubation period of years. CJD is believed to be caused by the same agent responsible for BSE. Both disorders are fatal brain diseases. The most common human form of CJD is now a variant called vCJD, not the classic form of CJD.

cross-contamination: The transfer of bacteria from food preparation surfaces, foods, hands, or utensils to another food. This is especially a problem with liquids from raw meat, poultry, and seafood, which can cause bacteria to contaminate foods or surfaces.

deficiency diseases: Diseases caused by poor nutrition and inadequate amounts of vitamins and minerals in the diet.

DNA: Deoxyribonucleic acid, a double-helix shaped molecule inside cells that carries genetic information.

Escherichia coli **O157:H7:** A bacterium, also known as *E. coli,* that can produce a deadly toxin. Symptoms include severe abdominal cramps, bloody diarrhea, and nausea. Sources of *E. coli* include undercooked or raw hamburger, uncooked produce, raw milk, unpasteurized juice, and contaminated water.

ethanol: Also known as ethyl alcohol, this substance can be used as an alternative fuel instead of gasoline. Easy to manufacture, it can be made from common crops such as corn and sugar cane.

ethylene: A gas used to make tomatoes ripen quickly.

fat-soluble vitamins: Vitamins A, D, E, and K, which are soluble in the fatty parts of plants and animals.

fertilizer: Natural or synthetic materials spread on soil to increase its capacity to support plant growth.

food additive: A substance added to foods to improve nutrition, taste, appearance, or shelf-life. In some instances, additives such as dyes or antibiotics have created food safety issues.

foodborne illness (also known as food poisoning): Infection caused by the transfer of microbial contaminants from food or drinking water. In most cases, the contaminants are bacteria, parasites, or viruses. The most commonly recognized infections are caused by the bacteria *Campylobacter, Salmonella,* and *E. coli.*

food inspection: The process of checking and ensuring that the nation's food supply is safe to eat and that proper sanitary conditions are enforced.

food poisoning: The common term for any illness caused by eating contaminated food. Food safety experts use the term "foodborne illness."

GLOSSARY

food safety: A system to ensure that illness or harm will not result from eating food. Everyone on the farm-to-table continuum, from production and processing to transportation, retail, or home, has an important role in keeping food safe.

Food Safety and Inspection Service (FSIS): The public health agency in the U.S. Department of Agriculture (USDA) responsible for ensuring that the nation's commercial meat, poultry, and egg products are safe, wholesome, and correctly labeled and packaged, as required by the Federal Meat Inspection Act, the Poultry Products Inspection Act, and the Egg Products Inspection Act.

gene: A section of DNA that carries instructions for a particular inherited feature such as hair color or height.

genetic engineering: The manipulation of genetic material to produce specific features in an organism.

genetically modified organism (GMO): An organism with new genetic material added to create desirable traits. This form of genetic engineering was made possible by the discovery of DNA and other scientific advances.

globalization: The development of a worldwide economic system.

Guillain-Barré syndrome: This disease affects the nerves of the body, beginning several weeks after diarrhea begins. It occurs when a person's immune system is "triggered" to attack the body's own nerves, resulting in paralysis lasting weeks, or sometimes longer. It is estimated that approximately one in every 1,000 reported cases of *Campylobacter* infection leads to this disease.

Hazard Analysis and Critical Control Point (HACCP): A science-based and systematic approach to prevent potential food safety problems, by anticipating how biological, chemical, or physical hazards are most likely to occur and by installing appropriate measures to prevent them.

herbicide: A chemical substance used to kill weeds or undesirable plants.

hygiene: Practices—such as cleanliness and maintenance of skin, hair, and nails—that promote health and prevention of disease.

infection: Attachment and growth of pathogenic microorganisms, including bacteria, viruses, and parasites, on or within the body of a human or animal.

insect resistance: The ability of some genetically engineered plants to make a substance that is poisonous to insects.

insulin-like growth factor: A substance called IFG-1, found in milk. Studies show that milk from cows treated with rBGH has higher levels of IFG-1, which may be associated with an increase in the rate of twin births.

irradiation: A process in which ionizing energy is used to kill pathogens and other harmful organisms in food by causing breaks in the DNA of the organisms' cells.

legumes: Considered the protein powerhouses of the plant kingdom, these plants have their seeds arranged in pods and include black, garbanzo, great northern, kidney, lima, mung, navy, pinto, and soy beans, as well as lentils and peas.

Listeria monocytogenes: Unlike most bacteria, this pathogen can grow slowly at refrigerator temperatures. It can cause serious health problems in vulnerable people, especially pregnant women, newborns, people with weakened immune systems, and the elderly.

malnourished: Lacking adequate nutrients in the diet.

malnutrition: The chronic lack of sufficient nutrients to maintain health.

microorganism: A microscopic life-form that cannot be seen with the naked eye. Types of microorganisms include bacteria, viruses, protozoa, fungi, yeasts, and some parasites and algae.

minerals: Inorganic substances that serve a function similar to vitamins. They include chemical elements such as calcium or iron, as well as some compounds.

mutation: An alteration in the hereditary material of a cell, which is transmitted to the cell's offspring. Mutations take place in the genes, which are segments of DNA molecules.

nervous system: The brain, spinal cord, and nerves that extend throughout the human body.

noroviruses: A group of viruses that affect the stomach and intestines. They are easily spread, and sources include raw oysters or shellfish, contaminated water, and person-to-person contact.

nutrients: Materials essential to the survival of an organism, including proteins, carbohydrates, lipids or fats, vitamins and minerals.

nutrition: The study of nutrients, their consumption, and how they are processed.

organic farming: A method of farming that does not use chemicals to kill weeds or pests.

parasite: An organism that feeds off of other organisms.

pasteurization: The process of destroying disease-causing microorganisms by heating food to a high enough temperature to kill the bacteria. The process was named for scientist Louis Pasteur.

pathogen: Any microorganism that is infectious or toxigenic and causes disease, including parasites, viruses, and some yeast and bacteria.

pesticide: A chemical used to kill plants or pests such as crop-damaging insects.

proteins: Large molecules essential to the structure and functioning of all living cells.

Pure Food and Drug Act: The passage of this act in 1906 allowed the government to gain control over impurities in food, drugs, and pharmaceuticals, and set up mechanisms for protecting the food supply. The Food and Drug Administration enforces this act.

recall: A voluntary action of removing a product from retail or distribution. The action is conducted by a manufacturer or distributor to protect the public from products that may cause health problems or possible death.

recombinant bovine growth hormone: A bovine growth hormone, made by genetically engineered bacteria, which is injected into cows to increase their milk production.

refrigeration: The process of chilling food for preservation.

Salmonella: A group of bacteria that cause fever, diarrhea, and abdominal cramps in a person from one to three days after the person eats contaminated food. Common sources include raw and undercooked eggs, raw meat, poultry, seafood, raw milk, dairy products, and produce. *Salmonella* can invade the bloodstream and cause life-threatening infections.

scurvy: A disease caused by a deficiency of vitamin C. Symptoms include a weakening of connective tissue in bone and muscle.

Shigella: This bacterium is carried only by humans, and causes diarrhea, fever, and stomach cramps starting a day or two after exposure. Poor hygiene, especially improper hand washing, causes it to be easily passed from person to person via food. Once the bacterium is in the food, it multiplies rapidly at room temperature.

Staphylococcus aureus: This bacterium is carried on the skin and in the nasal passages of humans. It is often found in infected cuts and burns; these wounds should always be covered with a water-proof bandage or plastic gloves to avoid contact with food. *S. aureus* produces a toxin that causes vomiting in as little as 30 minutes after ingestion. It also multiplies rapidly in food left out at room temperature.

sustainable agriculture: A method of farming designed to preserve the environment of the farm, livestock, and surrounding area while ensuring profitability.

toxin: A poison that is produced by a living organism.

transgenic organism: A genetically engineered animal or plant that contains genes from another species.

transovarian transfer: This occurs when certain pathogens, notably *Salmonella enteritidis,* infect the ovaries of hens and then infect the hens' eggs as they are being formed in the ovaries.

trichinosis: A parasitic disease caused by eating undercooked pork infected with a species of roundworm called the trichina worm. Symptoms include diarrhea, nausea, heartburn, and fever. Infection, once very common, is now rare in this country.

typhoid fever: A life-threatening illness caused by the bacterium *Salmonella typhi.* In the United States, about 400 cases are identified each year, and many are acquired while traveling internationally.

vegan: A vegetarian who does not consume any animal products and does not use products derived from animals, such as leather or fur.

vegetarian: A person who excludes all meat, poultry, and fish from his or her diet and instead eats plant foods. Some vegetarians include dairy products and eggs in their diets and are known as lacto-ovo-vegetarians; others who exclude all animal foods are known as vegans.

virus: A noncellular particle that consists minimally of nucleic acid (DNA or RNA) and protein. In order to survive, a virus must replicate inside another cell, such as a bacterium or a plant or animal cell.

vitamins: Organic substances essential to the nutrition of humans, animals, and some plants. Vitamins are needed in differing quantities. They work with enzymes in regulating metabolic processes.

water-soluble vitamins: Vitamins, such as vitamin C and the B-complex vitamins, that are soluble in the watery parts of plant and animal tissues.

Bibliography

Chapter One

"Adelle Davis, 1904–1974." In *Contemporary Authors Online*. Detroit: Gale Group, 2003. Reproduced in *Biography Resource Center* (Farmington Hills, MI: Thomson Gale, 2007). http://galenet.galegroup.com/servlet/BioRC (accessed September 19, 2007).

"Elmer Verner McCollum." In *Notable Scientists: From 1900 to the Present*. Detroit: Gale Group, 2001. Reproduced in *Biography Resource Center* (Farmington Hills, MI: Thomson Gale, 2007). http://galenet.galegroup.com/servlet/BioRC (accessed October 25, 2007).

"Frederick Gowland Hopkins." In *Science and Its Times*, vol. 6, *1900–1949*. Detroit: Gale Group, 2000. Reproduced in *Science Resource Center* (Farmington Hills, MI: Thomson Gale, 2007). http://galenet.galegroup.com/servlet/SciRC?ste=1&docNum=K2643412403 (accessed September 19, 2007).

"Frederick Gowland Hopkins." In *World of Biology,* online. Farmington Hills, MI: Thomson Gale, 2006. Reproduced in *Biography Resource Center* (Farmington Hills, MI: Gale, 2008). http://galenet.galegroup.com/servlet/BioRC (accessed September 18, 2007).

Hurley, Dan. *Natural Causes: Death, Lies, and Politics in America's Vitamin and Herbal Supplement Industry*. New York: Broadway Books, 2006.

"Johannes Baptista van Helmont." In *World of Chemistry,* online. Farmington Hills, MI: Thomson Gale, 2006. Reproduced in *Biography Resource Center* (Farmington Hills, MI: Gale, 2008). http://www.gale.cengage.com/BiographyRC/ (accessed September 18, 2007).

Kingsolver, Barbara, Steven L. Hopp, and Camille Kingsolver. *Animal, Vegetable, Miracle: A Year of Food Life*. New York: HarperCollins, 2007.

Nestle, Marion, and L. Beth Dixon. *Taking Sides: Clashing Views on Controversial Issues in Food and Nutrition*. New York: McGraw-Hill, 2003.
Smith, Jessie Carney, ed. *Notable Black American Women*. Detroit: Gale, 1992.
Toussaint-Samat, Maguelonne. *A History of Food*. New York: Barnes & Noble Books, 1998.
"Wilbur Olin Atwater." In *Dictionary of American Biography,* base set. American Council of Learned Societies, 1928–1936. Reproduced in *Biography Resource Center* (Farmington Hills, MI: Thomson Gale, 2007). http://galenet.galegroup.com/servlet/BioRC (accessed September 22, 2007).
Wiley, Harvey Washington. "The Next War." In *American Decades Primary Sources,* vol. 2, *1910–1919*, edited by Cynthia Rose, 466. Detroit: Thomson Gale, 2004.

CHAPTER TWO

Solorio, Season. "More Consumers Consider Themselves 'Regular' Supplement Users, Annual Survey Results Show." Washington, DC: Council for Responsible Nutrition, October 4, 2007. http://www.crnusa.org/prpdfs/CRN_PR_100407_ConsumerConfidence.pdf (accessed October 15, 2007).
U.S. Bureau of Labor Statistics. "Dietitians and Nutritionists." In *Occupational Outlook Handbook 2006–2007*. Washington, DC: Bureau of Labor Statistics, 2006.
"Vitamin." In *U-X-L Encyclopedia of Science*, vol. 9, *T–Z*, edited by David E. Newton, Rob Nagel, and Bridget Travers. Detroit: Gale, 1998.

CHAPTER THREE

"Borax Preservatives Found Injurious: Two Years' Test on Poison Squad Shows Anger in Canned Foods." *New York Times,* June 23, 1904, sec. 1: 9.
Davis, Carole, and Etta Saltos. "Dietary Recommendations and How They Have Changed over Time." In "America's Eating Habits: Changes and Consequences," edited by Elizabeth Frazao, special issue, *Agriculture Information Bulletin,* no. 750 (May 1999): 33–50. U.S. Department of Agriculture, Economic Research Service, Food and Rural Economics Division. http://www.ERS.USDA.gov/publications/aib750/aib750b.pdf (accessed September 18, 2007).
"Harvey Washington Wiley." In *Encyclopedia of World Biography,* 2nd ed. Detroit: Gale Research, 1998. Reproduced in *Biography Resource Center* (Farmington Hills, MI: Thomson Gale, 2007). http://galenet.galegroup.com/servlet/BioRC (accessed September 29, 2007).
Law, Marc T. "History of Food and Drug Regulation in the United States." In *EH.Net Encyclopedia,* edited by Robert Whaples. EH.Net, October 11, 2004. http://eh.net/encyclopedia/article/Law.Food.and.Drug.Regulation (accessed November 10, 2007).

"Poison Squad Escapes Federal Food Experts; Been Eating Doctored Food Five Months and Don't Like It." *New York Times,* May 22, 1904, sec. 1: 7.

Porter, Donna V. "Food Labeling Reform: The Journey from Science to Policy." *Nutrition Today* 28, no. 5 (October 1993): 7–13.

U.S. Food and Drug Administration. "FDA's Mission Statement." http:// www.fda.gov/opacom/morechoices/mission.html.

Weimer, Jan P. "USDA's Role in Nutrition Education and Evaluation." *Food Review* 18, no. 1 (January–April 1996): 41–46.

Chapter Four

Ackerman, Jennifer. "Food: Challenges for Humanity." *National Geographic* 200, no. 5 (May 2002): 2–51.

Adams, Jacqueline. "Holy Cow! What Now? Mad cow disease has hit the U.S. How worried should you be?" *Science World,* March 8, 2004.

Burros, Marian. "Eating Well: Questions on Irradiated Food." *New York Times,* October 15, 2003, sec. F: 6.

Center for Food Safety. "Food Irradiation." http://www.centerforfoodsafety.org/food_irrad.cfm (accessed April 14, 2008).

Centers for Disease Control and Prevention Food Safety Office. Web site home page. Updated January 19, 2009. http://www.cdc.gov/foodsafety/ (accessed March 22, 2009).

El Amin, Ahmed. "Irradiation Regulation Remains Inconsistent Worldwide." *FoodNavigator.com*, February 15, 2006. http://www.foodnavigator.com/news/printNewsBis.asp?id=65836 (accessed April 4, 2008).

Enis, Matthew. "FDA: New Irradiation Label Needed." *Supermarket News* 55, no. 16 (April 16, 2007).

"EU Lawmaker Says Irradiation Could Hide Rotten Meat." *Food Chemical News* 49, no. 30 (September 10, 2007): 13.

Evans, Christian. "FDA Plots to Dissolve Labeling Requirement for Irradiated Foods." *NaturalNews.com,* December 13, 2007. Reproduced by Organic Consumers Association. http://www.organicconsumers.org/articles/article_9072.cfm (accessed April 14, 2008).

"Food Additives Intended for Use in Processing of Canned Bacon: Proposed Revocations." *Federal Register* 33, no. 166 (August 24, 1968): 12055. Food and Drug Administration.

Food and Water Watch. "Irradiation: Expensive, Ineffective, and Impractical." http://www.foodandwaterwatch.org/food/foodirradiation/irradiation-facts (accessed April 16, 2008).

Gibbs, Gary. "Food Irradiation: The Untold Story." http://www.mindfully.org/Food/Food-Last-Forever-1.htm (accessed April 14, 2008).

Goldstein, Myrna Chandler, and Mark A. Goldstein. *Controversies in Food and Nutrition.* Westport, CT: Greenwood Press, 2002.

"Irradiation in the Production, Processing and Handling of Food." *Federal Register* 51, no. 75 (April 18, 1986): 13376, 13382. Food and Drug Administration; Department of Health and Human Services.

LaForge, John M. "Food Irradiation and Nuclear Weapons." *Z Magazine*, October 2000. http://www.zmag.org/zmag/viewArticle/13400 (accessed April 28, 2008).

LaForge, John. "Food Irradiation Is a Deal with the Devil." *Minneapolis Star Tribune*, February 3, 2001. Reproduced in *Common Dreams News Center*. http://www.commondreams.org/views01/0205-06.htm (accessed May 6, 2008)

Mead, Paul S., Laurence Slutsker, Vance Dietz, Linda F. McCaig, Joseph S. Breese, Craig Shapiro, Patricia M. Griffin, and Robert V. Tauxe. "Food-Related Illness and Death in the United States." *Emerging Infectious Diseases* 5, no. 5 (September–October 1999): 607–609.

Nestle, Marion. *Taking Sides*. New York: McGraw-Hill/Dushkin, 2003.

Nestle, Marion. *What to Eat*. New York: North Point Press, 2006.

Pauli, George H., and Clyde A. Takeguchi. "Irradiation of Foods: An FDA Perspective." *Food Reviews International* 2, no. 1 (1986): 79–107. http://www.cfsan.fda.gov/~acrobat/irrahist.pdf (accessed April 14, 2008).

"Policy for Irradiated Foods: Advance Notice of Proposed Procedures for the Regulation of Irradiated Foods for Human Consumption." *Federal Register* 46, no. 59 (March 27, 1981): 18992. Food and Drug Administration.

"Position of the American Dietetic Association: Food Irradiation." *Journal of the American Dietetic Association* 100, no. 2 (February 2000): 246–253.

Public Citizen. "History of Food Irradiation." http://www.citizen.org/cmep/foodsafety/food_irrad/articles.cfm?ID=1373 (accessed May 5, 2008).

"Report from the Commission on Food Irradiation for the Year 2005." *Official Journal of the European Union*, June 2, 2007: C 122/03. http://ec.europa.eu/food/food/biosafety/irradiation/index_en.htm (accessed May 15, 2008).

Steele, James H. "Food Irradiation: A Public Health Opportunity." National Foundation for Infectious Diseases, September 4, 1999. http://www.nfid.org/library/steele.html (accessed April 6, 2008).

"The Truth about Irradiated Meat." *Consumer Reports* 68, 8 (August 2003): 34–37.

U.S. Food and Drug Administration. "Irradiation of Food Packaging Materials." December 2007–January 2008. http://www.cfsan.fad.gov/~dms/irradrpt.html (accessed May 6, 2008).

World Health Organization. "High-Dose Irradiation: Wholesomeness of Food Irradiated with Doses above 10 kGy." Report of a joint FAO/IAEA/WHO study group, Geneva, September 15–20, 1997. Technical Report Series, no. 890: 161. Geneva: World Health Organization, 1997. http://www.who.int/ foodsafety/publications/fs_management/irradiation/en/ (accessed May 5, 2008).

CHAPTER FIVE

Becker, Geoffrey S., and Tadlock Cowan. "Agricultural Biotechnology: Background and Recent Issues." *Congressional Research Service (CRS) Reports and Issue Briefs,* September 2006: 4.

Center for Food Safety. "Genetically Engineered Food." http://www.centerforfoodsafety.org/geneticall7.cfm (accessed March 18, 2008).

Cornell Cooperative Extension's Genetically Engineered Organisms Public Issues Education (GEO-PIE) Project. "Genetically Engineered Foods: StarLink Corn in Taco Shells." New York: Cornell University, 2002. http://www.geopie.cornell.edu/educators/educators.html (accessed March 18, 2008).

Druker, Steven M. "A Report on the Results of *Alliance for Bio-Integrity v. Shalala, et al.*" Alliance for Bio-Integrity, October 1, 2003. http://www.biointegrity.org/report-on-lawsuit.htm (accessed March 19, 2008).

Fernandez-Cornejo, Jorge, and Margriet Caswell. "The First Decade of Genetically Engineered Crops in the United States." USDA Economic Information Bulletin, no. 11. USDA Economic Research Service, April 2006. http://www.ers.usda.gov/publications/eib11

Friedman, Lauri S., ed. *Genetic Engineering*. Farmington Hills, MI: Greenhaven Press, 2008.

Goldstein, Myrna Chandler, and Mark A. Goldstein. *Controversies in Food and Nutrition*. Westport, CT: Greenwood Press, 2002.

Hart, Kathleen. *Eating in the Dark: America's Experiment with Genetically Engineered Food*. New York: Pantheon Books, 2002.

Kanter, James. "EU Officials Propose Ban on Genetically Modified Corn Seeds." *International Herald Tribune,* November 21, 2007.

Lerner, K. Lee, and Brenda Wilmoth Lerner, eds. *Biotechnology: Changing Life Through Science*. Farmington Hills, MI: Thomson Gale, 2007.

Losey, John E., Linda S. Rayor, and Maureen E. Carter. "Transgenic Pollen Harms Monarch Larvae." *Nature* 399, no. 6733 (May 20, 1999): 214.

Meller, Paul. "Europe Rejects Looser Labels for Genetically Altered Food." *New York Times,* September 9, 2004.

Mellon, Margaret, and Jane Rissler. "Environmental Effects of Genetically Modified Food Crops: Recent Experiences." Paper presented by Margaret Mellon at "Genetically Modified Foods—the American Experience," sponsored by the Royal Veterinary and Agricultural University, Copenhagen, Denmark, June 12–13, 2003. Reproduced by Union of Concerned Scientists. http://www.ucusa.org/food_and_agriculture/science_and_impacts/impact_genetic_engineering/environmental-effects-of.html (accessed March 5, 2008).

Nestle, Marion, and L. Beth Dixon. *Taking Sides: Clashing Views on Controversial Issues in Food and Nutrition*. New York: McGraw-Hill, 2003.

Nestle, Marion. *What to Eat*. New York: North Point Press, 2006.

Pringle, Peter. *Food, Inc.: Mendel to Monsanto; The Promises and Perils of the Biotech Harvest*. New York: Simon & Schuster, 2003.

Rees, Andy. *Genetically Modified Food: A Short Guide for the Confused*. Ann Arbor, MI: Pluto Press, 2006.

Sample, Ian. "Biotech Firm Mans Barricades as Campaigners Vow to Stop Trials: Small Field Near Cambridge the Latest Battleground in Fight to Prevent GM Trials." *Guardian,* February 16, 2008: 6.

Simpkins, Jason, and William Patalon III, "Monsanto Reaps Huge Rewards from Its Blossoming Seed Business." *MoneyMorning.com*, January 7, 2008. http://www.moneymorning.com/2008/01/07/monsanto-reaps-huge-rewards-from-its-blossoming-seed-business/ (accessed January 7, 2008).

Smith, Jeffrey M. *Genetic Roulette: The Documented Health Risks of Genetically Engineered Foods*. Fairfield, IA: Yes! Books, 2007.

Thomson, Jennifer A. *Seeds for the Future: The Impact of Genetically Modified Crops on the Environment*. Ithaca, NY: Cornell University Press, 2007.

Torr, James D., ed. *Genetic Engineering*. Farmington Hills, MI: Thomson Gale. 2006.

Zied, Elisa, and Ruth Winter. *So What Can I Eat?! How to Make Sense of the New Dietary Guidelines for Americans and Make Them Your Own*. Hoboken, NJ: John Wiley & Sons, 2006.

CHAPTER SIX

"Americans Don't Make the Grade When It Comes to the ABCs of Nutrition and Multivitamins." *US Newswire*, December 13, 2007.

Barrett, Stephen. "How the Dietary Supplement Health and Education Act of 1994 Weakened the FDA." *Quackwatch.com*, February 2, 2007. http://quackwatch.com/02ConsumerProtection.dshea.html (accessed December 28, 2007).

Cheung, Thomas P., Charlie Xue, Kelvin Leung, Kelvin Chan, and Chun G. Li. "Aristolochic Acids Detected in Some Raw Chinese Medicinal Herbs and Manufactured Herbal Products: A Consequence of Inappropriate Nomenclature and Imprecise Labeling?" *Clinical Toxicology* 44, no. 4 (June 2006): 371–379.

"Dangerous Supplements: Still At Large." *ConsumerReports.org*, May 2004. http://www.consumerreports.org/cro.health-fitness/drugs-supplements-504 (accessed December 28, 2007).

Ernst, E., V. S. Vassiliou, J. P. Pelletier, D. O. Clegg, and D. J. Reda. "Glucosamine and Chondroitin Sulfate for Knee Osteoarthritis." *New England Journal of Medicine* 354, no. 20 (May 18, 2006): 2184–2185.

Gee, David. "The Sports Nutrition Explosion: The Changing Landscape of Sports Nutrition Market Is Filled with Controversy and Challenges, as well as Opportunities." *Nutraceuticals World* 9, no. 10 (November 2006): 38–42.

Goldstein, Myrna Chandler, and Mark A. Goldstein. *Controversies in Food and Nutrition*. Westport: Greenwood Press, 2002: 172–185.

Harris, Gardiner. "For FDA, a Major Backlog Overseas." *Virginian-Pilot*, January 29, 2008: 10.

Hurley, Dan. *Natural Causes: Death, Lies, and Politics in America's Vitamin and Herbal Supplement Industry*. New York: Broadway Books, 2006.

Jacobson, Michael F. "Supplement Scams." *Nutrition Action Healthletter*, September 2007: 2–11.

BIBLIOGRAPHY

Knight, Judson, and Neil Schlager. "Nutrients and Nutrition." *Science of Everyday Things* 3. Detroit: Gale, 2002.

Liebman, Bonnie. "Confusion at the Vitamin Counter: Too Little or Too Much?" *Nutrition Action Healthletter,* November 2007: 1–6.

"Linus Pauling." In *Scientists: Their Lives and Works*. Farmington Hills, MI: Thomson Gale, 2006. Reproduced in *Biography Resource Center* (Farmington Hills, MI: Thomson Gale, 2007). http://galenet.galegroup.com/servlet/BioRC (accessed December 21, 2007).

National Health Federation. "The NHF Declaration of Health-Freedom Rights." http://www.thenhf.com/declaration.htm (accessed March 22, 2009).

Nestle, Marion. *What to Eat*. New York: North Point Press, 2006.

"Robert C. Atkins." In *Biography Resource Center*. Farmington Hills, MI: Thomson Gale, 2008. http://galenet.galegroup.com/servlet/BioRC (accessed April 14, 2008). Originally published in *Newsmakers*, no. 2. Detroit: Gale Group, 2004.

Saul, Andrew W. "Vitamin Safety." *DoctorYourself.com.* http://www.doctoryourself.com/safety.html (accessed March 22, 2009).

Slutsker, Gary. "Killer Acids." *Forbes* 148, no. 5 (September 2, 1991): p. 144.

Solorio, Season. "More Consumers Consider Themselves 'Regular' Supplement Users, Annual Survey Results Show." Washington, DC: Council for Responsible Nutrition, October 4, 2007. http://www.crnusa.org/prpdfs/CRN_PR_100407_ConsumerConfidence.pdf (accessed October 15, 2007).

Stone, Irwin. *The Healing Factor: Vitamin C against Disease*. New York: GD/Perigee Books, 1972.

Swann, John P. "History of the FDA." U.S. Food and Drug Administration History Office. http://www.fda.gov/oc/history/historyoffda/fulltext.html (accessed December 1, 2007).

"Taking Too Many Multivitamins May Raise Prostate Cancer Risk." *Men's Health Advisor* 9, no. 8, August 2007: 6.

"Toxic Herb Sold via Internet." *Better Nutrition* 66, no. 1 (January 2004): 22.

Walsh, Nancy. "5-HTP Supplements Not Always Safer." *Family Practice News* 32, no. 19, October 1, 2002: 36.

Zelman, Kathleen. "The Truth behind the Top 10 Dietary Supplements." *Medicine Net.com*, August 24, 2007. http://medicinenet.com (accessed December 17, 2007).

CHAPTER SEVEN

American Cancer Society. "Cancer Prevention and Early Detection: Facts and Figures, 2007." Atlanta, GA: American Cancer Society, 2007. http://www.cancer.org/docroot/STT/content/STT_1x_Cancer_Prevention_and_Early_Detection_Facts__Figures_2007.asp (accessed May 20, 2008).

American Dietetic Association. "Position of the American Dietetic Association and Dietitians of Canada: Vegetarian Diets." *Journal of the American Dietetic Association* 103, no. 6 (June 2003): 748–765.

American Institute for Cancer Research. "Recommendations for Cancer Prevention." *AICR Diet and Health Guidelines for Cancer Prevention.* http://www.aicr.org/site/PageServer?pagename=dc_home_guides (accessed July 12, 2008).

Antrobus, Derek. "Philosophy of Diet or Philosophy of Life?" Paper presented at the 35th World Vegetarian Congress, July 8–14, 2002. Reproduced by the International Vegetarian Union. http://www.ivu.org/congress/202/texts/derek1.html (accessed July 12, 2008).

Barnard, Neal. "Meat's Striking Out." *USA Today,* May 21, 2008, sec. A: 11.

Brody, Jane E. "Final Advice from Dr. Spock: Eat Only All Your Vegetables. (Benjamin Spock recommends vegetarian diet for children)." *New York Times,* June 20, 1998, sec. A: 1.

"Dirty Birds: Even Premium Chickens Harbor Dangerous Bacteria." *Consumer Reports,* January 2007: 20.

Dowdle, Hillari. "Frances and Anna Lappé." *Vegetarian Times,* May 2008: 52–53.

Dworkin, Norine. "22 Reasons to Go Vegetarian Right Now: Benefits of Vegetarian Diet." *Vegetarian Times,* April 1999.

Goldstein, Myrna Chandler, and Mark A. Goldstein. *Controversies in Food and Nutrition.* Westport, CT: Greenwood Press, 2002.

Gorman, Peter. *Pythagoras: A Life.* London: Routledge & Kegan Paul, 1979.

Horsman, Jennifer, and Jamie Flowers. *Please Don't Eat the Animals: All the Reasons You Need to Be a Vegetarian.* Sanger, CA: Wood Dancer Press, 2007.

Kolata, Gina. "Vegetarians vs. Atkins: Diet Wars Are Almost Religious." *New York Times,* February 22, 2004, Week in Review: 12.

Lappé, Frances Moore. *Diet for a Small Planet.* New York: Random House, 1982.

Lappé, Frances Moore, and Joseph Collins. *Food First: Beyond the Myth of Scarcity,* Boston, MA: Houghton-Mifflin, 1977.

Lavelle, Marianne, and Kent Graber. "Fixing the Food Crisis." *U.S. News and World Report,* May 19, 2008: 36–42.

Miller, D. Patrick. "Frances Moore Lappé: Rediscovering America's Values." *East West,* September 1989: 26.

Murphy, Joan. "Chicken Industry Faults USDA Arsenic Study." *Food Chemical News* 45, no. 51, (February 2, 2004): 33.

O'Brien, Dennis. "Arsenic Used in Chicken Feed May Pose Threat: Hopkins Study Explores Risk to Consumers, Water." *Baltimore Sun,* May 4, 2004, sec. B: 1.

Pelton, Tom. "Arsenic's Use in Chicken Feed Troubles Health Advocates." *Baltimore Sun,* March 10, 2007, sec. A: 1.

Price, Lance B., Elizabeth Johnson, Rocio Vailes, and Ellen Silbergeld. "Fluoroquinolone-Resistant *Campylobacter* Isolates from Conventional and Antibiotic-Free Chicken Products." *Environmental Health Perspectives* 113, no. 5 (May 2005): 557–560.

SerVaas, Cory. "Diets that Protected Against Cancers in China." *Saturday Evening Post* 262, no. 7 (October 1990): 26–30.
Singer, Peter, and Jim Mason. *The Ethics of What We Eat: Why Our Food Choices Matter*. Emmaus, PA: Rodale. 2006.
Spencer, Colin. *The Heretic's Feast: A History of Vegetarianism*. London: University Press of England, 1995.
Spock, Benjamin. *Dr. Spock's Baby and Child Care*, 8th ed. New York: Pocket Books, 2004.
Stahler, Charles. "How Many Adults Are Vegetarian?" *Vegetarian Journal*, no. 4 (2006). http://www.vrg.org/journal/vj2006issue4/vj2006issue4poll.htm (accessed July 12, 2008).
Vesanto, Melinda, and Brenda Davis. *The New Becoming Vegetarian: The Essential Guide to a Healthy Vegetarian Diet*. Summertown, TN: Healthy Living Publications, 2003.
Wallinga, David. "Playing Chicken: Avoiding Arsenic in Your Meat." Minneapolis, MN: Institute for Agriculture and Trade Policy, 2006.
Whelan, Elizabeth M. "A Steak in Causing Cancer?" *Washington Times*, November 7, 2007, sec. A: 17.

CHAPTER EIGHT

Benbrook, Charles, Xin Zhao, Jaime Yanez, Neal Davies, and Preston Andrews. "New Evidence Confirms the Nutritional Superiority of Plant-Based Organic Foods." *Organic Center Critical Issue Report*, March 2008, 42. http://www.organic-center.org (accessed July 12, 2008).
Bowman, Cissy. "Harvey Case Tests National Organic Program." *Cooperative Grocer*, no. 118, May–June 2005.
Center for Food Safety. "Organic and Beyond." http://www.centerforfoodsafety.org/organic_an.cfm (accessed March 18, 2008).
Fromartz, Samuel. *Organic, Inc.: Natural Foods and How They Grew*. Orlando, FL: Harcourt, 2006.
Galbraith, Kate. "Beyond the Whopper: Fast Food Goes Organic and Natural." *Gristmill: The Environmental News Blog*. http://gristmill.grist.org (accessed July 10, 2008).
Goldstein, Myrna Chandler, and Mark A. Goldstein. *Controversies in Food and Nutrition*. Westport, CT: Greenwood Press, 2002.
Grandjean, Phillippe, et al. "The Faroes Statement: Human Health Effects of Developmental Exposure to Chemicals in Our Environment." *Basic and Clinical Pharmacology and Toxicology* 102, no. 2 (February 2008): 73–75.
Greene, Cathy. "Organic Labeling." In *Economics of Food Labeling*, Elise Golan et al., Agricultural Economic Report no. 793. USDA Economic Research Service, January 2001. http://www.ers.usda.gov/publications/ aer793/aer793g.pdf (accessed July 14, 2008).
Greene, Ward. "Guru of the Organic Food Cult." *New York Times Magazine,* June 6, 1971: 30–31, 54–60, 65–67.

Holden, Patrick. "Howard's Way." *The Ecologist* 31, no. 5 (June 2001): 30–36.
Kingsolver, Barbara, Steven L. Hopp, and Camille Kingsolver. *Animal, Vegetable, Miracle: A Year of Food Life*. New York, NY: HarperCollins, 2007.
Lawrence, Felicity. "Organic Milk Higher in Nutrients." *Guardian*, January 7, 2005: 10.
Lengeman, William I., III. "The Other Fast Food Nation: Organic Choices for People On the Go." *E Magazine* 18, no. 3. May–June 2007.
Mäder, Paul, et al. "Soil Fertility and Biodiversity in Organic Farming." *Science* 296, no. 5573 (May 31, 2002): 1694–1697.
Martin, Andrew. "Meat Labels Hope to Lure the Sensitive Carnivore." *New York Times*, October 24, 2006, sec. A: 1.
Minowa, Craig. "U.S. Government Facts: Children's Chemical and Pesticide Exposure via Food Products." Organic Consumers Association, July 2005. http://www.organicconsumers.org/organic/wic-faq.pdf (accessed May 20, 2008).
Mosteller, Rachel. "Thinking Globally, Eating Locally in the USA." *USA Today*, May 4, 2007, sec. D: 6.
"National Organic Program: Proposed Amendment to the National List of Allowed and Prohibited Substances." *Federal Register* 73, no. 135 (July 14, 2008): 40200. Food and Drug Administration.
Parks, Louis B. "Getting to the Root of the Issue: New USDA Labels Cultivate Recognition of Organic Industry." *Houston Chronicle*, October 13, 2002: 1.
Pennsylvania Department of Environmental Protection. "J. I. Rodale and Rodale Family: Celebrating 50 Years as Advocates for Sustainable Agriculture." PA Department of Environmental Protection, October 10, 1997. http://www.depweb.state.pa.us/heritage/cwp/view.asp?A=3&Q=444237 (accessed July 17, 2008).
Philpott, Tom. "The Case for Organic Builds." *Gristmill: The Environmental News Blog*. http://gristmill.grist.org (March 28, 2008).
Pollan, Michael. *The Omnivore's Dilemma: A Natural History of Four Meals*. New York: Penguin Press, 2006.
Posner, Joshua L., Jon O. Baldock, and Janet L. Hedtcke. "Organic and Conventional Production Systems in the Wisconsin Integrated Cropping Systems Trials: I. Productivity 1990–2002." *Agronomy Journal* 100 (2008): 253–260.
Rich, Deborah. "Not All Apples Are Created Equal." *Earth Island Journal*, Spring 2008. Earth Island Institute. http://www.earthisland.org/journal (accessed August 12, 2008).
Rodale, Ardath. "The Rodale Dream: 50 Years of Love." *Prevention* 52, no. 9 (September 2000): 275.
Schardt, David. "Organic Food: Worth the Price?" *Nutrition Action Healthletter*, July–August, 2007.
Schuett, Kathryn. "Organic Valley: Celebrating 20 Years of Doing Good and Doing Well." *Organic Processing Magazine*, May–June 2008. http://www.organicprocessing.com/magazine.htm (accessed August 4, 2008).

Welland, Diane. "Is It Safer to Eat Organic Spinach . . . or Peaches or Apples?" *Environmental Nutrition*, June 2007. http://www.environmentalnutrition.com (accessed June 12, 2008).

"When It Pays to Buy Organic." *ConsumerReports.org*. http://www.consumerreports.org/cro/food/diet-nutrition/organic-products-206/overview/index.htm (accessed July 12, 2008).

Chapter Nine

Ackerman, Jennifer. "Food: How Safe? How Altered?" *National Geographic* 200, no. 5 (May 2002): 2–51.
Altekruse, Sean F., and D. L. Swerdlow. "The Future of Foodborne Diseases." *Chemistry and Industry*, February 19, 1996: 132–136.
Bakalar, Nicholas. "Rise in Rate of Twin Births May Be Tied to Dairy Case." *New York Times*, May 30, 2006. http://www.nytimes.com/2006/05/30/health/30twin.html (accessed October 7, 2008).
Barone, Jennifer. "Milk Drinkers More Likely to Have Twins." *Discover* 28, no. 1 (January 2007): 48.
Baumler, Andreas J., Billy M. Hargis, and Renee M. Tsolis. "Tracing the Origins of *Salmonella* Outbreaks." *Science* 287, no. 5450 (January 7, 2000): 50–52.
Callaway, T. R., T. S. Edrington, R. C. Anderson, J. A. Byrd, and D. J. Nisbet. "Gastrointestinal Microbial Ecology and the Safety of Our Food Supply as Related to *Salmonella*." *Journal of Animal Science* 86, no. 14 (April 2008): E163–E172.
Centers for Disease Control and Prevention. "BSE (Bovine Spongiform Encephalopathy, or Mad Cow Disease." http://www.cdc.gov/ncidod/dvrd/bse (accessed September 23, 2008).
Dahl, Elizabeth, and Caroline Smith DeWaal. "Scrambled Eggs: How a Broken Food Safety System Let Contaminated Eggs Become a National Food Poisoning Epidemic." Center for Science in the Public Interest, May 1997. http://www.cspinet.org/reports/eggs.html (accessed October 23, 2008).
"*E. coli* Outbreak: Questions Loom on Food Safety." *Tulsa World*, September 4, 2008, sec. A: 14.
"FDA Strengthens Safeguards for Consumers of Beef: Issues Regulation on Animal Feeds with Added Safeguards Against BSE." *FDA News*, April 23, 2008. U.S. Food and Drug Administration. http://www.fda.gov/bbs/topics/NEWS/2008/new01823.html (accessed September 27, 2008).
"Fear of Fresh: How to Avoid Foodborne Illness from Fruits and Vegetables." *Nutrition Action Healthletter*, December 2006.
Hume, Scott. "Bush Boosts Food-Safety Budgets: Impact of Mad Cow Disease Incident Is Clear in Research and Testing Funds." *Restaurants and Institutions*, March 15, 2004: 60.
Martin, Andrew, and Griff Palmer. "China Not Sole Source of Dubious Food." *New York Times*, July 12, 2007, sec. C: 1.

Neergaard, Lauran. "The COOL Law: Country-of-Origin Labeling of Foods." *Virginian-Pilot*, September 30, 2008: 3.
Nestle, Marion. *Safe Food: Bacteria, Biotechnology, and Bioterrorism*. Berkeley, CA: University of California Press, 2003.
Nestle, Marion. *What to Eat*. New York: North Point Press, 2006.
Pampel, Fred C. *Threats to Food Safety*. New York: Facts on File, 2006.
Petersen, Melody, Christopher Drew, and Bud Hazelkorn. "New Safety Rules Fail to Stop Tainted Meat." *New York Times*, October 10, 2003, sec. A: 1.
"*Salmonella* Cases Exceed 1,000; FDA Unable to Pinpoint Source." *Virginian-Pilot*, July 10, 2008: 3.
Schmit, Julie. "U.S. Food Imports Outrun FDA Resources." *USA Today*, March 19, 2007, sec. B: 1.
Serrano, Alfonso. "How Safe Is Imported Food?" *CBSnews.com*, April 16, 2007 (accessed October 5, 2008).
Shin, Annys. "Does Ethanol Raise Risks?" *Washington Post*, November 4, 2008, sec. H: 1.
Sinclair, Upton. *The Jungle*. New York: Buccaneer Books, 1984.
Sylvester, Lisa. Interview by Lou Dobbs, *Lou Dobbs Tonight*. CNN, June 20, 2008.
U.S. Department of Agriculture Economic Research Service. "Food Illness Cost Calculator: *Salmonella*." http://www.ers.usda.gov/data/foodborneillness/salm_Intro.asp (accessed September 20, 2008).
U.S. Department of Agriculture Food Safety and Inspection Service. "Celebrating 100 Years of the Federal Meat Inspection Act (FMIA)." May 15, 2006. http://www.fsis.usda.gov/About_FSIS/100_Years_FMIA/index.asp (accessed September 21, 2008).
U.S. Food and Drug Administration National Advisory Committee on Microbiological Criteria for Foods. "Hazard Analysis and Critical Control Point Principles and Application Guidelines." Adopted August 14, 1997. http://www.cfsan.fda.gov/~comm/nacmcfp.html (accessed October 3, 2008).
U.S. Food and Drug Administration Center for Food Safety and Applied Nutrition. "Overview." http://www.cfsan.fad.gov/~lrd/cfsan4.html (accessed October 15, 2008).
"U.S. Food Safety in Question." *Medical Laboratory Observer* 39, no. 4 (April 2007): 15.

CHAPTER TEN

Belluck, Pam. "Obese Kids Show Early Signs of Heart Disease." *Virginian-Pilot*, November 12, 2008: 4.
Brownell, K. D. "Fast Food and Obesity in Children." *Pediatrics* 113, no. 1 (January 2004): 132.
Center for Science in the Public Interest. "Obesity on the Kids' Menus at Top Chains." August 4, 2008. http://www.cspinet.org/new/200808041.html (accessed November 5, 2008)

BIBLIOGRAPHY

Center for Science in the Public Interest. "California First State in Nation to Pass Menu Labeling Law." September 30, 2008. http://www.cspinet.org/new/200809301_print.html (accessed November 5, 2008).

"Cheeseburger Bill Puts Bite on Lawsuits." *CNN.com*, October 20, 2005. http://www.cnn.com/2005/POLITICS/10/20/cheeseburger.bill/index.html (accessed November 9, 2008).

Collins, Dan. "McDonald's Wins Fat Fight." *CBS News*, January 22, 2003. http://www.cbsnews.com/stories/2003/01/22/health/main537520.shtml (accessed November 9, 2008).

Gogoi, Pallavi. "From Fat Nation to Fit Nation: To Fight Obesity, the Government Should Boost Health Education and Help Shield Kids from Junk Food." *Business Week Online*, October 29, 2004. http://www.businessweek.com/bwdaily/dnflash/oct2004/nf20041029_8885_db045.htm (accessed November 11, 2008).

Gunderson, Gordon W. "The National School Lunch Program: Background and Development." USDA Food and Nutrition Service. http://www.fns.usda.gov/cnd/lunch/aboutlunch/programhistory_7.htm (accessed November 8, 2008).

Hellmich, Nancy. "Mothers Start a Food Fight." *USA Today*, August 8, 2007: D1.

Kingston, Anne, and Nicholas Kohler. "L.A.'s Fast-Food Drive-By: A City Council's Ban on Fast-Food Chains Is a Provocative Social Experiment." *Maclean's* 121, no. 33 (August 25, 2008).

Kummer, Corby. "Fat City." *Atlantic Monthly* 299, no. 2 (March 2007).

"L.A. Battles Tremors, Obesity: New Fast-Food Restaurants Banned in One Part of City." *Houston Chronicle*, July 30, 2008: 4.

Liebman, Bonnie. "The Changing American Diet: A Report Card." *Nutrition Action Healthletter* 29, no. 10 (December 2002).

Lopes, Gregory. "N.Y. Restaurants Cutting Trans Fat from Menus." *Washington Times*, December 6, 2006: C8.

Lubell, Jennifer. "Suit Alleges Junk-Food Brainwashing." *Pediatric News*, March 2006.

Lueck, Thomas J., and Kim Severson. "New York Bans Most Trans Fats in Restaurants." *New York Times*, December 6, 2006. http://www.nytimes.com/2006/12/06 (accessed November 9, 2008).

Maugh, Thomas H. "Link Found between Drinking Soda, Even Diet, and Disease." *Virginian-Pilot*, July 7, 2007: 5.

Muzaurieta, Annie Bell. "Are School Lunches Causing Childhood Obesity?" *TheDailyGreen.com*, November 3, 2008 (accessed November 3, 2008).

Physicians Committee for Responsible Medicine. "Healthy School Lunches: National School Lunch Program Background." http://www.healthyschoollunches.org/background/nutrition.html (accessed November 15, 2008).

Pollan, Michael. *The Omnivore's Dilemma*. New York: Penguin Books, 2006.

Roberts, Paul. *The End of Food*. Boston: Houghton Mifflin, 2008.

Schlosser, Eric. *Fast Food Nation: The Dark Side of the All-American Meal*. New York: Houghton Mifflin Company, 2004.

Schlosser, Eric, and Charles Wilson. *Chew on This: Everything You Don't Want to Know about Fast Food*. Boston: Houghton Mifflin, 2006.

Spake, Amanda, and Mary Brophy Marcus. "A Fat Nation." *U.S. News and World Report*, August 19, 2002.

U.S. Department of Health and Human Services Centers for Disease Control and Prevention. "Physical Activity and Good Nutrition: Essential Elements to Prevent Chronic Diseases and Obesity 2008." February 2008. http://www.cdc.gov/nccdphp/publications/aag/pdf/dnpa.pdf (accessed November 4, 2008).

INDEX

1906 Pure Food and Drug Act, 17, 20, 123–124, 149, 160–161, 191–192, 210
1938 Food Drug and Cosmetic Act, 21–22
1958 Food, Drug and Cosmetic Act, 33–34
Agriculture, Department of. *See* U.S. Department of Agriculture (USDA)
Aklylcyclobotanones (ACBs), 41
Alliance for Bio-Integrity, 57, 63
Alpha-tocopherol, 95–96. *See also* Vitamin E
American Cancer Society, 83
American Dietetic Association
　position on irradiation, 39–40
　and vegetarian diet, 77–78
　and vitamins, 65
American Heart Association, 77, 154
American Institute on Cancer Research (AICR)
　and vegetarianism, 83
American School Food Service Association (ASFSA), 153
Amines, 5
Amino acids, 11, 92, 207
Anaxagoras, 4
Animal agriculture, 84–88, 149–150
Animal and Plant Health Inspection Service (APHIS), 55, 125
　field trials, 55. *See also* U.S. Department of Agriculture (USDA)

Animal cruelty, 84–88
　and McLibel suit, 85
Anorexia, 98
Antibiotics, 89
　and livestock, 87–90, 128, 136
　and organics, 112–113
Aristolochia
　Chinese sales of, 72–73
　FDA action, 72
Arsenic
　and organics, 88–89
　in poultry, 88–89
Atkins, Robert C., 74
Atoms for Peace, 33, 129
Atwater, W.O., 7–8, 22,
　caloric tables, 7, 191
　farmer's bulletin, 22
Atwater-Rosa calorimeter, 7

B vitamins, 13–14, 67–68
Bacillus thuringiensis (Bt), 47, 132
　and corn, 47–48, 58, 61
Basic Four food groups, 23
Basic Seven Food Guide, 23. *See also* National Wartime Nutrition Guide
Bechler, Steve, 70
Becquerel, Antoine Henri, 32, 191
Beef
　and antibiotics, 87
　and bovine spongiform encephalopathy (BSE), 87–88, 128–129
　exports, 87–88, 129

Beef (*Continued*)
   feed, 87
   grass-fed, 15, 109, 112–113
   and hormones, 87
   production issues, 87–88
   recalls, 29, 88 (*see also* Bovine spongiform encephalopathy)
Beriberi, 5, 207. *See also* Nutritional diseases
Better School Food, 153–154
Botulism, 135–137, 208
Bovine growth hormone. *See* Recombinant bovine growth hormone (rbGH)
Bovine somatotrophin (BST)
   ban, 87
   in dairy cows, 87
Bovine spongiform encephalopathy (BSE), 31, 43, 87, 193, 207
   cases in U.S., 60, 137–138
   feed guidelines, 59–60, 128–129
   and genetically modified organisms, 59–60, 131–132
Bryant, A.P., 7–8
Bureau of Animal Industry Act, 122
Bureau of Foods Irradiated Food Committee (BFIFC)
   and the IFTG, 36
   recommendations, 35–36

Caffeine
   in sports drinks, 67
   U.S. intake levels, 67
Calcium, 7, 67
   absorption of minerals, 96
   osteoporosis, 96
   vegetarian sources, 96 (*see also* Dietary supplements)
Calgene, 53–54
   lawsuit by Monsanto, 54
Caloric tables, 7. *See also* Atwater-Rosa calorimeter
Calories, 3, 154, 194
   measurement of, 6 (*see also* Metabolism)

Campbell, T. Colin, 84
Campylobacter, 207
   and grass-fed beef, 109, 112
   and Guillain-Barrè syndrome, 90, 136
   and irradiation, 31, 129–131
   symptoms of, 90, 135–136
Cancer
   and pesticides, 111
   U.S. statistics, 77
   and vegetarian diet, 77, 83–84
Carbohydrates, 207
   complex, 12, 93
   simple, 12, 93
   sources of, 11–12, 92–93
Carson, Rachel, 101
Cattle. *See* Beef
Center for Consumer Freedom (CCF), 91
Center for Food Safety, 39, 57, 63, 193
   and Harvey, Arthur, 105–106
   and Public Citizen, 39
Center for Food Safety and Applied Nutrition. *See* U.S. Food and Drug Administration (FDA)
Center for Foodborne Illness Research and Prevention, 133–135
Center for Science in the Public Interest (CSPI), 22, 77, 133–134, 147
Centers for Disease Control and Prevention (CDC), 18, 29, 119–120, 135, 138, 151
Charles, Prince of Wales, 61, 193
Cheeseburger bill. *See* Personal Responsibility in Food Consumption Act
Chemical additives, 22, 144
   and FDA, 18
Chicken, 139
   animal cruelty, 85–86
   and arsenic, 88–89
   avian influenza, 124

consumption, 89
country-of-origin labeling, 126
egg safety, 85–86, 121–125
free-range, 109
inspection methods, 124
Poultry Products Inspection Act (PPIA), 124
processing, 85–86
production guidelines, 85–86
China, 84, 121, 126. *See also* Melamine
China study, 84. *See also* Campbell, T. Colin
Cholesterol, 9, 12, 94, 146
Chondroitin, 68
Chromium, 96–97
Civil War, 7
Collins, Joseph
Institute for Food and Development Policy, 82
and Lappe, Frances Moore, 82
Colman, Norman J., 18
Combs, Susan, 153
Commonsense Consumption Act of 2007, 155. *See also* Personal Responsibility in Food Consumption Act.
Community Health Councils (CHC), 147
Community supported agriculture programs (CSA), 118
Consumer Federation of America, 133
Consumers Union, 127, 133
Copper, 97
and zinc, 97
Coulee Region Organic Produce Pool (CROPP), 107
Country-of-origin labeling (COOL), 126–128
Council for Responsible Nutrition (CRN), 13, 66, 74
and antibiotics, 87
and bovine somatotrophin (BST), 87
dairy cows, 86–87
milk production, 87
survey results, 66–69
Creutzfeldt-Jakob disease. *See* Variant Creutzfeldt-Jakob disease (vCJD)
Cross-contamination, 31, 139–140, 208
Cross-pollination, 50, 62
Curie, Marie, 32
Cyclospora parasite, 138

Davis, Adelle, 8–9
Diabetes, 148, 151, 155
Dietary Guidelines for Americans, 23–25, 94–95, 165–168, 194
and school lunches, 152
and vitamins, 65–66
dietary recommendations, 84, 94–95
Dietary Reference Intakes (DRI), 23, 94–95, 152
Dietary Supplement Health and Education Act (DSHEA), 69, 193
and ephedra, 70
Dietary Supplement and Non Prescription Drug Consumer Protection Act, 70–71
Dietary supplements, 13
government regulations, 69–71
and L-tryptophan, 71–72 (*see also* Vitamins; Supplements)
Division of Chemistry, 18–19. *See also* U.S. Food and Drug Administration (FDA)
Drucker, Stephen M., 63

Earthbound Farm, 106–107
and bagged lettuce, 106
spinach recall, 114
E-coli, 30, 128, 208
CDC estimates, 119–120, 135–136
and grass-fed beef, 109, 112
and irradiation, 38

E-coli (*Continued*)
   Jack in the Box, 121–122, 127, 135
   and organic food, 114
   spinach recall, 38, 114
   symptoms, 90, 136
Edible Schoolyard Project, 153
Egg safety, 121–125
   in Europe, 85
   free-range, 109
   product guidelines, 86
   and salmonella, 124–125, 194
Eijkman, Christian, 5, 191
Eisenhower, Dwight David, 33, 129, 192
Electron beam radiation, 30–31
Elixir Sulfamilamide
   1937 tragedy, 21, 192
   FDA reaction, 21
Environmental Protection Agency (EPA), 54
   and arsenic, 88
   GMO regulations, 54–56
   and pesticides, 111
Environmental Working Group (EWG)
   and pesticides, 116–117
Ephedra
   classification, 70
   FDA ban, 70–71, 194
European Commission (EC), 41–42, 58, 130
European Consumers Organization (BEUC), 41
European Union
   common catalog, 58
   egg production guidelines, 86
   and GM seeds, 50
   hog production guidelines, 86
   import bans, 57–59

Fast food, 143–156
   economics of, 143–144
   in schools, 152–153 (*see also* Junk food)

Fast food restaurants
   bans, 145–149
   and diabetes, 148, 151, 155
   and legislation, 145–149, 194
   and obesity, 147–148, 150–151, 155
Fats
   and cholesterol, 93–95
   Dietary Guidelines for Americans, 94–95
   and hydrogen atoms, 12, 94
   monosaturated, 12, 94
   plant sources, 93–94
   saturated, 12, 94
   in school lunches, 152–153
   unsaturated, 12, 94
Feed additives, 87–90
Federal Farm bill, 110
Federal Meat Inspection Act (FMIA), 123–124, 149, 191
Fertilizer
   chemical, 101, 113, 149, 208
   and soil quality, 102, 113
Fiber, 93
Fish oil, 69
FlavrSavr tomato
   and Calgene, 53–54
   FDA ruling, 53, 193–194
   and Monsanto, 54
Folic acid
   and birth defects, 14, 68
   and cancer, 75
   effects of, 14, 68
   government policy, 68
Food and Drug Administration (FDA)
   Bureau of Science, 35
   Center for Food Safety and Applied Nutrition, 125–126
   history of, 18–19, 192
   Produce Safety Action Plan, 128
   role in food regulation, 18–19, 68, 89, 123, 125, 129–131
   substantially equivalent designation, 53–54
Food and Water Watch, 38

Food desert, 147
Food First. *See* Collins, Joseph; Institute for Food and Development Policy; Lappè, Frances Moore
Food guide pyramid. *See* U.S. Department of Agriculture (USDA), food guide pyramid
Food irradiation
   cross-contamination, 31–32
   effects on foodborne diseases, 30–32
   FDA approval of, 33–37, 192–193
   fuel sources, 30
   safety issues, 129–131
   and U.S. Army, 42–43, 193
   U.S. statistics, 119–120 (*see also* irradiation)
   USDA regulations, 33–35
Food labels, 20–22, 55–56, 127
   and organics, 108–110
Food rationing, 23
Food recalls, 57
   beef, 29, 88
   statistics on, 119–120, 125 (*see also* Food safety)
Food safety, 119–142, 178–182, 192, 209
   and Hazard Analysis and Critical Control Point Program (HACCPP), 127–128, 182–185
   imports, 120–121, 126
   inspections, 123–124, 126
   labels, 192
Food Safety and Inspection Service (FSIS). *See* U.S. Department of Agriculture (USDA)
Food scientists, 15
Foodborne diseases, 29–30, 135–138, 178–182, 208
   and country-of-origin (COOL) law, 126. *See also* Food safety
Foot and mouth disease, 100–101
   British epidemic, 100

Frankenfood, 46
Franklin, Benjamin, 79–80
Free-range eggs. *See* Egg safety
Fructose, 12
Funk, Casimir, 5

Gamma ray irradiation, 30–31
Gene flow, 48
Generally recognized as safe (GRAS), 55–57, 192
Genetic engineering (GE), 45–64, 209
   attacks on, 58–59
   cross-pollination, 48
   and France, 58–60
   moratorium, 58–59, 61
   seeds, 52 (*see also* Genetically modified food (GM))
Genetically modified food (GM), 45–64, 193, 209
   and BST, 87
   critics of, 38–39, 62–63, 131–132, 193
   in Europe, 57–61, 194
   health risks, 50–51, 131
   labels, 62–64
Genetically modified organism (GMO), 45–64
   DNA changes, 46–47
   effects on insects, 48
   labels, 55–56
   and organic crops, 104 (*see also* Genetically modified food (GM))
Glucose, 12, 96
Glucosamine, 68
GM Watch, 63
Goodman, Drew, 106–107
Goodman, Myra, 106–107
Graham, Sylvester, 80–81
Grandjean, Philippe, 111
Gray (gy), 31. *See also* Rad
Great Depression, 110
Greenpeace, 105
   policy on GMOs, 63–64
Guillain-Barrè syndrome, 90, 136, 209

Hahnemann, Dr. Samuel Christian Friedrich, 68
  and homeopathy, 68
Halloran, Jean, 127
Harvey, Arthur, 105–106, 194
  lawsuit, 105–106
Hazard Analysis and Critical Control Point Program (HACCP), 127–128, 182–185, 194, 209
Health and Human Services. *See* U.S. Department of Health and Human Services (HHS)
Help International Plant Protein Organization (HIPPO), 83
Hemoglobin, 11
Hemolytic uremic syndrome, 121, 138
High fructose corn syrup, 144, 150
High-density lipoprotein (HDL), 9
  effects on health, 12, 146. *See also* Cholesterol
Hippocrates, 4, 10
Hog production, 86
  government moratorium, 86
Homeopathic medicine, 68
Hopkins, Frederick Gowland, 5
Howard, Sir Arthur, 100–101
  and soil nourishment, 100–101
Human Nutrition Information Service (HNIS), 22
Hunt, Caroline, 23
Hydrogen peroxide, 37
Hydrogenation, 12–13

Industrial Revolution, 149
Institute for Agriculture and Trade Policy (IATP), 88
Institute for Food and Development Policy, 82
International Atomic Energy Association (IAEA), 40. *See also* Joint Expert Committee on Food Irradiation
International Food Information Council (IFIC), 10, 39
International Irradiation Association, 39
International Society for Orthomolecular Medicine (ISOM), 66, 73. *See also* Pauling, Linus
Ionizing radiation, 30
Iron, 96
  vegetarian sources of, 96
Irradiated Foods Task Group (IFTG), 36. *See also* Bureau of Foods Irradiated Food Committee (BFIFC)
Irradiation, 29–43, 129–131, 171–176, 209
  beef, 103–131
  and the European Union, 41–42
  herbs and spices, 36
  labels, 34–35, 41–42, 103–131, 192
  lettuce and spinach, 131
  mutations, 38, 130–131
  opponents of, 37–39, 130
  and organics, 104
  pork, 35–36, 130, 191
  vitamin loss, 38
  waste, 43

Jack in the Box. *See* E. coli
Joint Expert Committee on Food Irradiation, 40
Junk food, 144
  and advertising, 146–147
  school bans, 146–147(*see also* Fast food)

Kalafa, Amy, 153
Kittrell, Flemmie Pansy, 8, 192
Kowalcyk, Barbara, 135

L-tryptophan
  ban, 51, 71, 193
  eosinophilia myalgia syndrome, 71
  and GMOs, 70

tragedy, 50–51, 71–72 (*see also* Dietary supplements)
Labels. *See* Nutrition Fact Label
Lacto-ovo-vegetarian, 78. *See also* Vegetarian
Lappè, Frances Moore, 82, 192
  and Collins, Joseph, 82
  Institute for Food and Development Policy, 82
Liberia, 8
Lincoln, Abraham, 18, 79, 122, 191
Lind, James, 5, 191. *See also* Scurvy
Listeria, 135–136, 209. *See also* Foodborne diseases
Los Angeles, 145–149, 194
Low-density lipoproteins (LDL), 9, 12
  effects on health, 146

Mad cow disease. *See* Bovine spongiform encephalopathy (BSE)
Magnesium, 97
Mallon, Mary, 123–124. *See also* Typhoid Mary
Malnutrition, 101
Manganese, 97
Mason, Dr. Joel, 75
  and folic acid, 75–76
McCollum, Elmer, 6–7
McDonalds, 143–144, 154–155, 192
  McLibel suit, 85
Meal replacements, 67
Meat
  associated medical costs, 120
  consumption, 77, 80
  exports, 122
  health risks, 90–91
  inspection, 122
Meat Inspection Act. *See* Federal Meat Inspection Act (FMIA)
Medwatch, 76
Melamine, 121. *See also* China

Mendel, Lafayette Benedict, 6
Metabolism, 6
Minerals
  and calcium, 96
  major, 14, 96
  nutritional aspects of, 96–97, 210
  trace, 14, 96
Monarch butterfly, 48–50. *See also* Genetic engineering (GE)
Monsanto
  early GMO development, 47–50
  FlavrSavr tomato, 53–54, 193–194
  lawsuits, 50, 133
  profits, 61–62
Multivitamins, 66–67. *See also* Dietary supplements
MyPyramid, 25. *See also* U.S. Department of Agriculture, food guide pyramid

Nader, Ralph, 37, 134. *See also* Public Citizen
National Academy of Sciences
  Institute of Medicine, 111, 146–147
National Aeronautics and Space Administration (NASA). *See* U.S. National Aeronautics and Space Administration
National Association of Anorexia and Associated Disorders, 98
National Cancer Institute, 77, 111
National Cattlemen's Beef Association (NCBA), 91
National Center for Complementary and Alternative Medicine, 68
National Center for Food and Agriculture Policy (NCFAP), 62
National Chicken Council, 85, 89
National Climate March, 82–83, 194
National Food Irradiation Program, 33
National Foundation for Cancer Research, 75

National Health Federation (NHF), 66
National Institute of Health (NIH), 18, 68, 88
National Labeling and Education Act (NLEA) of 1990, 13, 22
National Organic Program (NOP), 105
National Organic Standards Board (NOSB), 104–105
National Pork Producers Council (NPPC), 91
National School Lunch Program, 151–153, 185–187, 192
National Wartime Nutrition Guide, 23. See also Basic Seven Food Guide
Nestle, Marion, 154
Nixon, Richard, 151, 192
Noroviruses, 135–137, 210
Nutrients, 6. See also Nutrition
Nutrigenomics, 4, 9–10
Nutrition, 3
   and genes, 9–10
   definition of, 11, 210
   theories of, 6–7
   labels, 22
Nutrition Business Journal, 65–66
Nutrition Fact Label, 13, 22, 168–171, 193
Nutritional genomics, 4, 9–10
Nutritional deficiencies, 6–7
Nutritional diseases
   beriberi, 5
   obesity, 147–148, 150–151
   rickets, 6–7
   rodent studies, 6–7
   scurvy, 5

Obesity, 3, 144–145, 147–148, 150–151
Omega-3 fatty acids, 112
   American Heart Association recommendations, 69
   health benefits, 69

Organic Consumers Association, 38, 105
Organic Farming and Gardening Magazine, 101, 106
Organic food
   and fast food, 115–116
   federal subsidies, 110
   history, 100–103
   nutritional advantage, 113–114
   and pesticides, 111 (*see also* Organics)
Organic Food Production Act of 1990 (OFPA), 64, 104–105, 193
Organic labels, 108–110
Organic Trade Association (OTA), 106, 113
Organic Valley,
   company goals, 107
   and Wal-Mart, 108
Organics
   crop yields, 114–115
   federal standards, 104
   labels, 108–110, 176–177
   sales figures, 99, 103
Organization for Economic Cooperation and Development (OECD), 83
Osborne, Thomas B., 6
Overnutrition, 151, 154
Ovo-vegetarian, 78. See also Vegetarian

Pauling, Linus, 68, 73–75
   and vitamin C, 68
People for the Ethical Treatment of Animals (PETA), 82–85
   and global warming, 83
   National Climate March, 82–83
Perry, Jan, 146
Personal Responsibility in Food Consumption Act, 155
Pesca-vegetarian, 78. *See also* Vegetarian
Pesticides
   and children, 111–113

insect resistance, 112
in milk, 112
and organic farming, 113–114
U.S. usage, 112, 149, 192
Pigs, 86
Plant-based diet. *See* Vegetarian
Poison squad, 19–20, 123
Pollo-vegetarian, 78. *See also* Vegetarian
Polychlorinated biphenyls (PCBs), 64, 88, 109, 128
Potassium, 97
Poultry Products Inspection Act (PPIA), 124. *See also* Chicken
Prescott, Samuel, 32–33, 191
Processed foods, 149–151
Protein
complementing, 92
excess, 92–93
sources of, 11, 92–93
Proxmire, William, 72, 193
Public Citizen, 37, 133–134
and Center for Food Safety, 99
Pure Food and Drug Act. *See* 1906 Pure Food and Drug Act
Pusztai, Arpad, 60–61, 194
Pythagoras, 79

Rad, 31. *See also* Gray (gy)
radiation, 29–43
uses of, 31
Radiolytic product (URP), 36
Recombinant bovine growth hormone (rbGH), 109, 210
effects on fertility, 132–133
Recombinant DNA (rDNA), 46
Recommended Dietary Allowances (RDA), 23, 73, 92, 192. *See also* Reference Daily Intakes (RDI)
Reference Daily Intakes (RDI), 23, 91–92, 194
Registered dietitian, 15
Rickets, 6–7. *See also* Nutritional diseases

Rodale, Jerome Irving, 101–103
Roosevelt, Franklin D., 21–22
support of RDA's, 23, 123
Rosa, E.B., 7
Roundup, 47, 61–62. *See also* Monsanto
Rubin, Susan, 153

Safe Tables Our Priority (STOP), 131, 135
Safety, food. *See* Food safety
Salmonella, 30, 38, 138, 211
1994 ice cream outbreak, 124–125, 141
2008 pepper outbreak, 120–121, 141
CDC estimates, 119
economic cost, 120
in eggs, 124–125
and farming practices, 124–125
symptoms of, 90, 135–136
Sarkozy, Nicholas, 58, 194
Saturated fats, 12–13, 93–95
Schizophrenia, 9
Schwarzenegger, Arnold, 145
School lunch program. *See* National School Lunch Program
School Meals Initiative for Healthy Children, 152
Scurvy, 5, 211
and vitamin C, 5 (*see also* nutritional diseases)
Selenium, 75, 97
and diabetes, 76
FDA recommendations, 76, 97
Sense about Science, 62
Shigella, 31, 135–137, 211
Siemon, George L., 107
Sinclair, Upton, 19, 122, 142, 191
Sodium, 144, 150, 152
U.S. intake levels, 67
Soft drinks, 154
Soil and Health Foundation, 101
South Korea, 87–88, 129
Spencer, Collin, 79

Spock, Benjamin, 84
  vegetarian diet, 84
Sports nutrition supplements
  caffeine content, 67
  sodium content, 67
  sports drinks, 67
StarLink corn, allergic reactions, 52, 131–132
  class action suit, 56–57
  recall, 51–52, 194
Stone, Irwin, 74
  and Linus Pauling, 74–75
Subsidies, 110
Supplements. *See* Dietary supplements
Szent-Gyorgyi, Albert, 75
  and Pauling, Linus, 75
  and vitamin C, 75

Tesco, 148–149
Thiamine, 5. *See also* Vitamin B
Trans fats
  bans, 146
  health effects of, 13, 94–95, 146
  and nutrition labels, 22, 94, 194
  (*see also* transfatty acids)
Transfatty acids, 13, 94. *See also* trans fats
Truth about Trade & Technology, 62
Tryon, Thomas, 79
Turner, Matthew, 148
Two Angry Moms, 153–154. *See also* Kalafa, Amy; Rubin, Susan
Typhoid Mary, 123–124
Tyson Foods, 89–90, 127

Union of Concerned Scientists, 48, 63
United Egg Producers, 86
United Nations Food and Agricultural Organization (FAO)
  report on irradiation, 40–41
U.S. Army Food Irradiation Program, 33

U.S. Atomic Energy Commission, 33
U.S. Department of Agriculture (USDA)
  Animal and Plant Health Inspection Service (APHIS), 54–55
  Bureau of Animal Industry, 122
  Dietary Guidelines for Americans, 23–25
  Economic Research Service, 120
  food guide pyramid, 24–25, 97–98, 187–189, 193
  Food Safety and Inspection Service (FSIS), 34, 89, 94, 122–125, 129–131, 193, 209
  history of, 17–18, 122–124, 191
  role in food regulation, 17–18, 123–125
  Office of Experimental Stations, 7, 22
  school lunch program, 152–153
U.S. Department of Health and Human Services (HHS), 77, 111
  food regulation, 17–18
  National Center for Health Statistics, 22
U.S. Food Safety and Inspection Service (FSIS), 34, 89, 94, 122–125, 129, 138–139. *See also* U.S. Department of Agriculture (USDA)
U.S. National Aeronautics and Space Administration (NASA), 127, 130

Van Helmont, Johannes Baptista, 4
Variant Creutzfeldt Jakob disease (vCJD)
  link to bovine spongiform encephalopathy, 60, 87, 138
  (*see also* bovine spongiform encephalopathy)

INDEX

Vegan, 78–79, 211. *See also* Vegetarian
Vegan Society, 83
Vegetarian
  and anorexia, 98
  celebrities, 78
  fats, 93–95
  health effects, 78–98
  history, 79–83
  and pesticides, 88
  and protein, 92–93
  statistics, 78
  types of, 78–79, 211
  vitamin B12 deficiency, 91
  vitamins and minerals, 95–97
Vegetarian Resource Group (VRG), 78
Veneman, Ann, 105
Vitamin A, 6
  sources of, 13–14, 95
  and vegetarians, 95 (*see also* Vitamins)
Vitamin B, 6
  sources of, 13–14
  and vegetarians, 95–96 (*see also* Vitamins)
Vitamin B-12, 5–7
  deficiencies, 68, 91, 95
  and DNA, 91
  recommended levels, 91
  sources of, 13–14
Vitamin C, 14, 68
  sources of, 95 (*see also* Vitamins)
Vitamin C Foundation, 66
Vitamin D, 74
  and calcium, 67–69, 95
  deficiencies, 7
  sources of, 13–14, 95–96 (*see also* Vitamins)

Vitamin E, 13–14, 112
  fat soluble, 95–96
  study results, 96
  vegetarian sources, 95–96 (*see also* Vitamins)
Vitamin K, 13–14, 96
Vitamins, 65–76
  B12 deficiency, 68, 91, 95
  deficiencies, 7
  and dietary supplements, 13
  evidence of health benefits, 75, 95–96, 113
  fat soluble, 5, 13, 95–96, 208
  sales figures, 65
  sources of, 13–14, 95–96
  vegetarian intake, 95–96
  water soluble, 5, 13, 95–96, 212
Von Liebig, Baron Justus, 6, 101
Von Mayer, Julius Robert, 6

Wal-Mart, 107–108, 117
Water, 14–15
Waters, Alice, 153
Webster, John, 85
Whole Foods, 99, 115–117, 148–149
Wiley, Harvey Washington, 19–20, 123, 134, 191. *See also* Poison squad
World Cancer Research Fund (WCRF), 83
World Health Organization, 138
  and irradiation, 40
  and PETA, 83
World Trade Organization, 58, 193
  EU ban, 58

X-ray radiation, 29–31
X-ray technology, 31, 191

Zinc, 97

ABOUT THE AUTHOR

Sharon Zoumbaris has worked as a professional librarian, school librarian, freelance writer, and storyteller. She is the co-author of *Teen Guide to Personal Financial Management* (Greenwood, 2000), *Food and You: A Guide to Healthy Habits for Teens* (Greenwood, 2001), and *Encyclopedia of Diet Fads* (Greenwood, 2003).